Voices From Far Away

Steve Rhodes

Contents

Author's Introduction

The book that you are holding in your hands took a long time to write. Almost a lifetime in fact. That it has been a well-lived one, and hopefully far from over yet, is something that I am fairly proud of. Well, so far anyway. I am 59 years old as I write this introduction, and at times, still struggling like a bastard just to keep my head above water. One of the key reasons for that struggle is that I am still coming to terms with - and in some ways recovering from a disease called Autoimmune Encephalitis (Type LGI1).

If you are wondering what that is, well, it is a condition in which the body's immune system attacks the brain, causing inflammation. The immune system produces substances called antibodies that mistakenly attack healthy brain cells. Not good eh? There are many different types of AE as I will abbreviate it from here on in, if that's okay with you? Saves on the typing, and the constant use of spellchecker. The LGI1 thing is just the specific cells in the brain, so is the specific type of AE that gave me a run for my money.

It first raised its ugly head in early to mid 2018 and towards the end of that year I was admitted to hospital. I was, over a period of nearly five and a half months, transferred another two times to alternative hospitals for different types of treatment, care or rehabilitation. I was finally discharged from the last one around the middle of March 2019. A not inconsequential amount of that final stay was spent just sitting on a general ward simply waiting for the next treatment to either start, or in some cases finish.

I believe that this book is a 'must read' for anyone who has ever experienced a long-term, or life-altering illness that may have a connection to the brain, or to the immune system...but I am not suggesting that you read it if only those elements apply. It is essentially a book about my journey, and a disease that is so little-known by the general populace that I believe there is a need for more to be written about it to raise its profile. Perhaps in doing so it will also give a boost to the organisations that support it around the world.

This book has been on Amazon for over two years now in a more generalised format, as initially it was a full autobiography that covered many other aspects of my life, and what makes me tick as a human-being. It sold a few copies to some friends and acquaintances, for which I am very grateful, but not enough however. Not by a long shot. The book contains some really important messages in my opinion as the disease (AE) is very, very hard to diagnose if certain tests are not undertaken. The result therefore is that people have symptoms (and myriad ones at that) that get treated...but very often the 'whole picture' is not seen, or not present in those early stages, and therefore the specific cause of the malaise remains hidden.

So here I am splitting the original autobiography in half, so that it focuses almost solely on the illness, tests, diagnosis, treatments, discharge, and the final return home. I figured that I might as well start at the beginning (where else) where there were only signs (or symptoms) that something was wrong and the visits to the GP - to try to work out exactly what was going on, reference to the drugs and advice taken at each step, and the complexity of finding out what the actual cause for all of this was.

There are ensuing chapters that cover the hospital visits, the final admission and the time spent in the first hospital where I went downhill pretty rapidly. I have also given detail of the measures that had to be put in place to keep me safe whilst there and the eventual diagnosis - which very likely saved my life. Then the book talks a little more about the treatments, visits, assessments and the like.

There is naturally a chapter that talks about my final discharge home where the journey really started...all over again in some ways. Maybe not so much the actual 'being at home' per se, but more to do with not feeling like the same person I had been prior to AE, and not knowing where on earth I fit in anymore.

In truth I have often felt that I simply don't. Not anymore anyway...but let's cover that later on eh?

The final chapters talk about a relapse, which started just over a year ago now and has resulted in visiting more hospitals, specialists, and clinics throughout 2021. I went through another full round of highly exhaustive blood tests, psych evaluations, brain and body scans, to try to get to the bottom of the issue. It was triggered by a huge return of the absences, or seizures and boy did they come armed with reinforcements!

And whilst I would love to tell you that following all of the tests they found something substantial or treatable, they didn't. But maybe more on that later on too eh?

You may note that I often refer to life as a journey. I strongly believe that it is. And a bloody challenging one at that...at times! There will be many storms along the way. Some of them big and potentially dangerous. But there will also be days or weeks when the sun will come out and the sea will be calm. Then you get to lie up on the deck and enjoy the warmth, and the sun's rays on your skin. Maybe you'll get to dive off the boat and swim for a while in the clear blue waters.

The storms though...they are never very far away. This book is the story of a survivor. And one day I hope to take real pride in being that person, as I have often wondered if there is anything good about me at all. Truth!

The feelings that were lost to me over those first two months I am experiencing for the very first time.

So forgive the odd smeared and blurred line or word, as they will be where my tears landed. It is February 8th, 2020 (at the time that I wrote that line) and I have been unwell for about two years now.

Maybe I should start at the beginning though...

The Beginning

Towards the middle of 2018 I started to feel 'kind of different.' A little 'out of sorts,' if you will. I know that neither statement is very accurate, enlightening or revealing, but it was all I had at the time. The symptoms were really subtle and all quite commonplace viewed as a singular complaint, or malaise. On their own, they could have been seen simply as the result of stress or a 'normal' pressured life, the loss of a loved one, a change in a weather pattern, or a change of circumstances. I found myself getting headaches, tiredness, and bouts of nausea, disrupted or irregular sleep patterns, disturbing dreams, and more.

Close friends and colleagues tell me that I was behaving 'oddly' at work too. Hard to quantify, but it is amazing how much we are able to dismiss, but in hindsight think 'yeah, there were a lot of things that did not make sense.' Hindsight is a beautiful thing eh?

I'm afraid that had I not found a journal that I was keeping at the time, I would not have been able to piece together the signs that I had the onset of a brain disease, which I, like most people had never even heard of: AE. It is basically an inflammation of the brain tissue and apparently, the most common cause is viral infections. In rare cases, it can be caused by bacteria or even fungi, but enough of the medical science and 'proper' terms just now. Let's get back to the story eh?

In the middle of October (the 15th to be precise), last year, I was taken to Guildford Hospital by a colleague as she, like many of my friends and co-workers, became highly concerned that my behaviour had rapidly become very bizarre indeed. She told me that I turned up at her office to 'train' her staff on a computer system. Yet there was no such training booked or even scheduled.

It also seems that I had started to obsess about work, and if you knew me at all, that would make very little sense indeed and many people since the beginning of my recovery have commented on this. I myself have even expressed incredulity, as whilst I like and enjoy my work, it sure does not define me in any way, shape, or form.

What I do love is: travelling, socialising (the introvert's version anyway), movies (not cinema), listening to, collecting, playing, and writing music. I play acoustic and electric guitar and can bluff some keyboards and drums too. Oh, and since it turns out that with practice and persistence that I can also hold a note, I now adore singing too! There is nothing more energising and 'releasing' than singing at the top of your lungs. Swear to God!

I used to love reading and the reason I say, 'used to love' is, that reading has become one of quite a number of activities I cannot abide now. I have tried, and can still get through a book if it is very moving and not too long. On a bad day, I will struggle to select a piece of music that I can tolerate, only to rush back into the lounge seconds later to turn it off. AE does some odd things to a person's previous likes, dislikes, tastes, and personality. You better believe it.

I cannot tell you anything more about the end of 2018 as I have absolutely no recollection of it or my time in Guildford hospital. Pretty much from the beginning of October until the end of December 2018 my memory has been wiped clean. I don't recall a single worker's face, name, or the names of either of the two wards that I was on. All of that now resides in the 'Dead Zone' as I now call it.

I have since visited Guildford Hospital on one occasion, with my friend Lisa. Quite a few of the nursing and ward staff recognised me on entering one of the wards that I was in. They made quite a fuss of me and there were some lovely hugs too. For me, it was all pretty weird and not just a little overwhelming as they clearly liked me, and were delighted to see me walking, talking, and pretty much lucid. As lucid as I ever was, or will be.

Whilst I was there, I apparently underwent a huge battery of tests. All of which came out clear, negative, or inconclusive. This is apparently quite typical of Encephalitis (type LGI1) as it is very hard to diagnose. I lost around 11 kilos in weight over the first two months, which I sure can't stand to lose as I am hardly carrying a spare pound from all the exercise that I do. Oh, and as time went on, I slept a LOT, which I understand is the natural way for our bodies to fight infection.

I cannot recommend highly enough that we listen to our bodies. Quite why we seem to ignore the hammering on the door, that it gives us when we overdo the alcohol, or eat way too much, or stop going to the gym, I have no idea. I guess it is simply that those things are 'easy.'

I ask you this though; should life be easy? I admit that I have tried but failed, on many occasions to listen to my inner voice, but it sounds way too much like the Darkman. So, I fight (or fought at least) the perceived limitations that I have as a human. I guess I am a painfully slow learner. Some might say an idiot!

My close friend Lisa (guardian angel) tells me my friends and colleagues visited in their droves in the first two months in

Guildford hospital – a fact that still moves me to tears. Apparently, I kept running away in the first few weeks. I have to say that I rather like that story as not many people could catch me or keep up for the distance I could/can run.

The hospital had to find a lawful way of keeping me in the hospital due to my 'diminished capacity,' so they applied for a DOLS (Deprivation of Liberty Safeguard). Lisa recently showed me my paperwork that kept me in place and reading it was NOT easy. That belongs in capital letters due to the sheer weight of understatement inherent in it.

I re-read it just last Saturday and it resulted in my being absolutely distraught. Unsurprising really as it was terrifying and moving in equal measure! That this person, who was miles (light-years) from sanity, self-awareness, ability to perform even the simplest of tasks, personal care, etc. was me...well, I am almost lost for words to describe it.

I have contacted my friend and ex-colleague on the DOLS team to ask if I can include it here in this book as it was so moving. I think it has to be seen. I am going to share it with some of my friends too, as I feel that it is key to my making as full of a recovery as I can. Frankly, it is a miracle that I am living alone, independent in all tasks, able to walk, talk, work, run, etc. I am a fucking walking miracle!!

The hospital had to find a solution to my wandering and running away in that first month, so they stationed a big, male guard on my ward. I will find out his name and let you all know. My friend told me that one of the 'guards' kept falling asleep and I love that one time it happened the hospital called Lisa and informed her that I had disappeared again. She found me down the road waiting at the bus stop. I like that story. It still makes me smile to this very day, as I have always done random things to confuse and hopefully amuse myself and other people.

Lisa also tells me that I deteriorated pretty quickly and that one time when she visited she found that the curtains were drawn around my bed. The doctors and nurses looked pretty concerned, as they were unable to rouse me. I had been sleeping most of the time over a fair period of weeks and at that point, my friends were all pretty convinced that I was never going to regain my sanity, as when they visited I either talked nonsense, or about work, or slept, or said very little. Oh, and for a while, I apparently talked so quietly that it was quite hard to hear me. Not a trait that I am known for, for sure!

I don't recall anything at all. I was truly lucky however and responded well to the risky course of treatment that the doctors decided to go with as a final act of desperation, which was pretty much 'kill or cure' at that time. This is also documented in the DOLS paperwork, so maybe I am making that the next chapter. Anyway, timely treatment is absolutely key to a successful, and/or fuller recovery from AE.

I 'came to' and after just a few days I was able to recall my name and now, with a hopefully firm diagnosis, it was the job of the hospital to determine how seriously I had been affected in other areas. There can be any amount of impairment to a persons' faculties as a result of this disease, depending on things like: age, fitness, duration of inflammation, severity, and the time taken to diagnose and treat. After some time I was transferred to a stroke/rehabilitation unit in Woking. I was considered to be stable enough to be moved at that point.

Once again, I don't recall anything about that time, or the transfer at all.

Towards the end of December, I regained more cognitive functions and memory. I would love to say that I enjoyed my time in Woking hospital – which is a weird term to use for a hospital stay - but I felt it to be completely inappropriate for me, as a previously very fit human. I retreated into fairly angry sullen silence for pretty much the whole time that I was there.

That I had lost my ability to run any kind of distance and was skin and bone was anathema to me. I hated it! Luckily, I was once again able to read books, which has always been a lifelong passion for me, and that allowed me to spend many, many hours just sitting around, supposedly 'getting better.'

In the first month or so in Woking I was offered Gym sessions which I also hated as they were aimed at people who had experienced strokes and were trying to regain the use of limbs, or re-learning walking, balance, or weight-bearing. None of this seemed relevant to me and I found it humiliating. In truth, I started to find even those sessions tiring. I have never told anyone that. Truth.

Sometimes, when I asked to go outside (the one place that I thrive and adore completely) a worker would have to accompany me, for a simple run or walk around Woking Park. The months in bed on one ward or another, had robbed me of any muscle tone that I had prior to becoming unwell, and I was sickened by what had become of me. It was truly shocking to find that two laps (sometimes only one) around a small, winter-frozen park in ugly old Woking would tire me out completely. Good food and ammunition for the ever-growing inner critic eh?

Again, humiliation visited me (frequently) and I was angry, and I guess not always the easiest person to be around. I felt hollow and 'fake'. That last sentence is kind of hard to explain and saddens me no end. I felt like I was trying to convince these strangers that I used to have boundless energy, strength, and vitality.

It felt hollow coming out of my mouth like I was now some sad, lost soldier wearing his war medals to feel like he used to 'be someone,' but now he is just another lonely old man staring into the past. In truth I always felt – and still do to this day in some ways - that they probably thought I was full of shit and just making it up. How could it come to this?

I pulled away even further. I spoke less and less at mealtimes. Not that anybody seemed to notice or care anyway. I sat and moodily listened to a handful of the older male patients as they would hold forth for the billionth time about one achievement of theirs or another. They seemed (to me at least) to drone on ceaselessly about themselves.

I believe that to be a very typical male trait. At least in my experience of many blokes. As soon as I had finished my meal I would get up and leave the dining room, often without saying anything at all. I was enormously grateful for having my own room away from everybody I can tell you.

Note - to (an awful lot of) males – try to catch yourself next time you find yourself talking at people and not listening to the person, or 'persons' standing, or sitting in front of you.

Focus and perhaps even pay closer attention and you will notice just how bored or uncomfortable they look. Stop talking! Battle for some self-awareness. It is worth it.

Those two months or so, in Woking were (or at least felt at the time) interminable. I am almost grateful that the memories that I have of it are now vague and misted like the cracked, dusty windows in an old deserted warehouse. The staff there though were amazing and very patient. Well, they would have to be, to put up with me. It is important for me to acknowledge all the time and energy that everyone put in. Even if I was busy pulling further and further away.

I was doing my best at the time to connect with assessors and professionals, who were trying to gauge the overall effects on my remaining faculties and abilities. My writing had become a spidery scrawl, which filled me with shame, disgust, and anger. My mathematical and problem-solving skills were really poor at first. Let us note, just for the record however, that I have always been utterly shit at anything to do with numbers. Perhaps as a result of childhood teaching experiences, or just because of who I am. So no real surprises there.

What nobody could take into account is my personality and life experiences. You see, I hate to be put on the spot! When I feel watched, my interior critic screams at me at the top of his lungs *"NO GOOD"* so when I am under any kind of 'spotlight' it is so hard to focus. I literally feel the eyes of the person, or persons, in front of me burning into me and agreeing with my big, fat, lazy but oh so observant inner critic, and all I can hear and process is white noise. Fact!

I have always been that way, to some degree, and that goes way back to being five years old. During my first few weeks in my primary school, a Mathematics teacher singled me out and pulled me to the front of the class to explain to the class the meaning of Binary. I had no idea. He employed shouting at me as his skilled 'teaching style'. To my mind, to this very day, I cannot shake the notion that it is the Teacher that should do the teaching, not the kids. Their job is learning. Anyone else confused about that?

I wish so much that I could have looked up at him and said *"I'm five years old sir. So, I am coming at this for the very first time! Maybe once I have learned this stuff, then we can discuss the meaning of things, and whilst we are at it, the need for shouting."* But who is ever that smart or precocious when a class full of eyes and ears are trained on you? And at five years old.

Now though...all these years later, I was being told some areas of my brain may take months, or years to repair and that I just needed to be patient. All I really wanted was for someone to let me go home. Odd isn't it...that we call people in hospitals Patients? It has never, ever occurred to me to wonder where, or when the term was first coined. I know I could look it up in the blink of an eye...but where is the fun in that? I sure understand it now. Five months in hospital and trust me....it is the only term that fits.

But I digress. Again.

One morning around mid-February 2019 I was informed by nursing staff or the consultant (I don't fully recall now) that I was to be transferred to Tooting Hospital in London. I think I had barely finished breakfast when they told me to pack my things and that sometime during the day I would be picked up.

Now, we all know that things in hospitals can move pretty slowly, so I packed my few, meagre belongings into a couple of bags and perched on the end of my bed, relieved to be leaving. I don't recall if I was reading anything at the time. I think I had all but given up by that time. I had been lent so many books by friends by that point, it's pretty hard to remember.

Within an hour, three red-faced ambulance crew members came rushing into my room to find a bored and to all intents and purposes, pretty healthy-looking male sitting on his hospital bed. They were slightly annoyed as they had apparently been given the impression that I was an emergency.

I didn't even need to sit in a wheelchair to walk out back to the waiting ambulance, though I dimly recall that I was told/asked to. Not sure about that detail. The blue light was switched off and I sat in the back with two of the crew whilst we twisted and turned our way into London. What I am very sure about, however, is that I said goodbye to not one of the other patients. Charmer huh? That journey to Tooting seemed to last forever.

I spent just under a month in Tooting hospital and in that time received a number of treatments aimed at targeting the specific symptoms of my 'brand' of AE. I know that I underwent two rounds of Plasma exchange where essentially the blood is removed, cycled out of the body, washed to remove damaging antibodies, and returned. That treatment takes about three hours. The whole time, you have to sit, pretty still, and simply breathe. In, and out again. You can read and such....but I found it hard to. Again, the nursing staff were amazing. Truly amazing.

Since leaving Tooting Hospital I have also had a set of chemotherapy treatments. Six to be precise, over a three-month time period, but maybe we will talk a little more on that later on though. I am not going to list and describe all the types of AE or the ways in which it can be transmitted (or 'triggered') as I have no intention for this to be an academic piece of writing.

Besides which, the first friend to read an initial draft said, *"what is the point or focus of this book Steve? The bits about your life are, however, amazing."* I rather agreed with her. With the availability of information on the Net now, you can find out for yourself if you are concerned or interested enough. If you have any of the early traits that I describe at points throughout this book, however, PLEASE do read up, or talk to your GP. Quickly.

My friends tell me that I was unnaturally patient throughout my time in all three hospitals, but really, I was not feeling that much, emotionally. No. That was to come later. In my time in Tooting, I completely gave up reading. I just lost all interest. It didn't matter what the topic of the book was. Instead, I took to people watching, sleeping, and simply sitting on my bed staring out at the grey London skyline.

At the time of writing this sentence my love of reading hasn't really returned. I just can't find the desire to read, whether it is fact or fiction. It is fortunate that I enjoy writing now and I am loving writing this book!

I felt quite numb to be honest and in some ways that allowed me to tolerate being told when treatments were delayed or outright cancelled, and that we would start afresh next week, which meant another interminable weekend whiling my time away on a hospital ward. Watching paint dry is more interesting. I swear to God!

My friends continued to visit me regularly, and that in all truth, is pretty much the only thing that kept me going. Without friends I fear that I would sink without a trace. Lacking family is a hard to quantify 'space' to occupy. Hard to explain to others anyway. It is a feeling of not really being anchored anywhere. Easy to just drift away, and end up far from the shoreline and hopelessly lost out at sea.

What I did learn (step-by-tiny-step), is just how much I mean to my friends, but more on that later on. Maybe. So they would turn up at St George's Hospital in Tooting, and we would simply up and disappear, off to dinner, or to the pub, or for a walk, and return to the ward later; without even telling anyone where we were going, or when we would be back.

I got told off by the nurses a few times for doing that. Which was pretty fair play I would say. Yes, I did start telling them after a while but that could result in being told 'no' and that, on occasions, seemed trickier and less palatable to me than simply 'swanning off.'

I do need to say this though (again) and this comes from the bottom of my heart; the nursing staff in every one of those hospitals were incredible! We DO NOT pay enough respect to the health system in the UK. Not even close. Go to Tooting Hospital at any time of the day, or night and walk the corridors, the wards, and car parks. The sheer volume of people moving through those hallways will take your breath away.

End of memory

March 2018

This was a notable date only as it was the first entry in a Positivity Journal that a Canadian friend of mine encouraged me to keep. I figured that as I spent a lot of 2018 trying to develop gratitude (never a bad thing), for all the good things in my life, that it should go in here.

I know it is not an original idea by any means but as my language and writings, songs, etc. up to that point are all pretty bleak (some say negative), it sure seemed like a good idea and something that might help me grow.

There were clearly some early signs that all was not well health-wise in those journals. I have spoken to people since I was discharged from hospital to get an even wider picture. Like people at work, friends, and medical staff, they all said there were things that seemed small at the time, but that they just figured it was me being 'different.'

The below are some extracts from journals and diaries that I was keeping at the time and they clearly refer to some symptoms that could have flagged up the onset of the disease too. Bear in mind throughout this book however that diagnosing AE is difficult and you HAVE to be actively looking for it to spot it.

Monday July 16th, 2018.

- I feel a little out of sorts
- I feel like there is a 'storm' coming
- Quite tearful when watching Ally McBeal - the childhood scenes are upsetting me. Very deeply

I know what you might be thinking - "does he really like Ally McBeal?" Well the truth is, I really do. It might not be entirely cool but that is no longer something that I worry about. Why the hell should I? Culturally the English are noted for their lack of emotion, or lack of touch, or displays of affection. I want nothing to do with any of that! I eschew any definitions or labels as to whom I choose to be. That is and always has been anathema to me.

Tuesday 21st August 2018.

- So, I need to reflect a little here, as the first few weeks have been uncomfortable, but surely showing me things.

- Sadness/tearfulness
- Some anger and frustration
- Some fear (following the recent little health concerns)
- I have also found myself wanting to be away from my house. Being indoors troubles me in ways that are not clear to me. I have at times felt 'too alone' and have wanted/needed something or someone, to fill the space.

Wednesday 22nd August 2018.

- I haven't mentioned that I have been having some 'weird spells' of nausea over the last week or so. It would be fair to say that it has me scared. I don't know what is wrong, but I now feel vulnerable. Not a great feeling...but boy, does it make me grateful for all the good health that I have always experienced?

Sunday 9th September 2018.

- My health seems to be slowly returning so am grateful there (ironic entry)
- There is some movement in my emotional wellbeing too though I am very tearful. Go figure

Monday 10th September 2018.

- A pleasing day at work
- The blood test is pretty clear
- Chinese medicine theories are helping me to 'take part' in some minor ways in getting my health back on track

Sunday 16th September 2018.

- Nearly a month since my weird 'health issues' started
- I really want to understand the underlying causes and will try to be mindful and aware
- The symptoms have now abated to a low-grade set of 'nervous waves' that come and go throughout the day
- The visual disturbances have gone, which is a step in the right direction and as I write this, I am in Cap Feret way down in the south of France, not too far from Biarritz. As always, it is beautiful!

December 2018

Today I pulled out all the diaries and writing books that I have kept over the last two years or so. I want to try to piece together all the bits that I have forgotten about of the last two months of 2018. Unsurprisingly for the months of October and December, there is nothing. I have no recollection of my two months in Guildford Hospital at all. For that detail, you will need to read my friend Lisa's story. She wrote it a few weeks back, and it has been submitted for approval to the Encephalitis Society who will consider it to go onto their patient's stories pages on their website. As it is coming up for World Encephalitis Day they are heavily entrenched in fundraising and TV campaigns. So it came at just the right time.

Anyway, I got to the very slim black diary which has simply 18/19 on the cover in large, shiny writing. I had pulled out most of the pages, as I did not want reminders of all the days at home just sleeping and trying to fill time. I found that I could not look at them. I seem to have left all the pages from 23rd December 2018, some pages of January, February, and up to March. The below extract comes from that diary.

March 8th, 2019

I noted that all the entries in December are written in Lisa's handwriting. She would write down all the people who were visiting me and at what time etc. It breaks my heart in two, that I was not only that lost but also that someone cared that deeply for me. I am also humbled by it. There are some entries that I cannot look at as they are written in a spidery scrawl. The writing of someone that I cannot face fully at the moment. Well, not without crying a lot. Mind...I have been doing that a fair bit of late, anyway.

January 26/27th 2019

- I have been allowed a rare home trip for Saturday and Sunday.
- Returned to the unit in the afternoon.

My mood has been pretty low over the weekend. I was not as 'up' being at home, as I had expected and hoped I would be. It served more, as a reminder of all that has happened over the last four months, and all the things that I have had to cope with. It also makes me realise how far I still have to go, to return to some kind of 'stable' life again.

February - Friday 15th 2019

- I got whisked over to St George's Hospital in Tooting today. Not unexpected but when it happened it sure was rushed

March - Tuesday 12th 2019

- I was discharged home today

I turn to Kate Bush here (who I consider to be pretty much an utter genius) to make an awe-inspiring level of sense of the lives of some people who don't see that really talking and really feeling is the definition of really living. And it has no shame attached to it at all. Why would it? Oh, I nearly forgot to mention that it is about being a man, and feeling left out and helpless after the birth of a child.

> *"All the things I should have said, but I never said*
> *All the things I should have done but I never did.*
> *All the things that you wanted for me.*
> *Give me these moments back."*

Kate Bush – *This Womans' Work*

I co-run a men's support group now with Paul (a close friend of mine) and it strikes me almost every single week that we all seek some kind of meaning in (or to) life. Yet with so little time, that seeking can become a distraction from truly living and simply being grateful for everything around us. The older I get, the more I am convinced that there is no reason for living. No purpose. It is simply to be lived...and lived fully!

> *"Without understanding how vulnerable and fleeting this all is We risk being and feeling only half alive for our entire lives*
> *And that is the very definition of sadness".*

Steve Rhodes – *The Foolish and the Fleeting*

Steve's story (from the outside)

This chapter was written by Lisa Mallet, a very close friend who looked after me when I was lost to AE – type LGI1. People like Lisa are few and far between. She is a rare combination of humble, happy, non-judgemental, and has an incredible inner strength and determination that I am profoundly grateful to have experienced, and learned from...I hope.

Summer to October:

Looking back now, there were signs from as early as July 2018 that something was wrong. Steve had completed a half marathon on a hot day and, in the weeks afterward, he started to describe his calf muscles as feeling like a 'bag of snakes' – they were constantly twitching (fasciculation).

He reported vivid dreams and problems sleeping. He was uncharacteristically stressed about his work as a trainer for Social Services. The first symptoms that sent him to his GP were dizziness and nausea. He then started complaining of a strange sensation in his chest which he found difficult to describe. He said it was quite a pleasant feeling as if something exciting was going to happen.

The GP did blood tests and checked out his heart which were all normal. He was prescribed Propranolol for anxiety and a sleeping tablet.

October 2018 – Sudden memory loss

One Tuesday evening, I came home from work to two confused messages on my answerphone from Steve. I called him to see what the messages were about, but Steve could not remember leaving them. I went over to his house. He was about to eat his dinner uncharacteristically early. He wasn't aware of what time it was and could not tell me what he had done that day. He didn't know if he had been to work or not.

On the advice of 111, I took him to the hospital. He underwent a CT scan of his head which was negative and blood tests which were all normal. He underwent a thorough physical examination and was seen by the on-call psych team. As a stroke and a brain tumour had been ruled out by the scan, the working diagnosis was anxiety.

The Doctor wanted to admit Steve for further tests but he refused to be admitted and so he was discharged home with an urgent referral to the local mental health team. Over the next few days, his behaviour varied from relatively normal to strange. His memory seemed back to normal.

Occasionally, he would stutter and turn his head to the right, usually if he was talking about work. I accompanied him to see his GP. A couple of times in the waiting room, he shouted out random words. His strange behaviour worried the GP and we agreed that I would take his car keys off him. She got on the phone and chased the referral to the mental health team.

A couple of days later, I was woken by Steve at my front door. It was 3am, dark outside and he was wanting his car keys to drive to work. Steve prides himself that he can guess the time correctly to within 15 minutes. That day (and for about two months afterward) he could not tell the difference between 3am or 3pm.

I took him back to his house and installed myself on his sofa which is where I spent the next few nights until he was admitted. He was barely sleeping, and if he did, he physically acted out his dreams during which he was training people. Writing this it seems so obvious that there was something seriously wrong. However, at the time his symptoms were transient and variable. The side effects of the medication he was on included paranoia, confusion, memory loss, and peculiar mannerisms. Investigations had been normal.

Mid October – Admission to hospital

A week after his first visit to A&E, Steve was back there again following strange behaviour at work. He underwent yet more tests. After several hours and more examinations, I was told that the most likely diagnosis was dementia. Then there was a breakthrough – a positive test. His sodium levels were too low (hyponatremia). I was relieved to hear that this was treatable and could be the cause of his symptoms. He was admitted. Treatment involved restricting his fluids over a number of days. Steve underwent more scans to rule out a tumour (which can cause sodium ion imbalance).

At this stage, Steve was permanently confused. He knew that he was in the hospital, but thought he was there assessing the staff. Initially, there was some improvement as Steve's sodium balance returned to normal but then his symptoms worsened again.

He was restless, still not sleeping, and would wander around the ward. He refused to put his things in the locker by his bed and he always had his bag packed ready to go.

In the first week, he went missing twice from the ward, trying to make his way back home. After the second escape attempt, he was put under a DOLS (Deprivation of Liberty) for his own safety. This meant he had a staff member permanently assigned to him. In the first few days of having one-to-one nursing, his allocated staff member would be exhausted trying to keep up with Steve's wanderings.

Now that his sodium levels were normal there was no obvious reason for the symptoms to continue. The working diagnosis returned to anxiety and I was told that the next day he would be sectioned. However, the next day, nearly two weeks after being admitted, Steve had an EEG which showed that he was having seizures. The strange grimacing and arm movements turned out to be facial brachial seizures. This was followed by an MRI which showed inflammation on his brain. He had encephalitis.

At this point, the most likely diagnosis was AE as other types of encephalitis were ruled out with blood tests. We waited weeks for his autoimmune screen to come back from Oxford which was positive for the LGI1 antibody.

Meanwhile, Steve continued to deteriorate. I had to take his mobile phone off him as he was calling friends in the middle of the night confused. He became sleepier and weaker. He lost 11 kilos of muscle and could no longer stand for more than a couple of minutes.

Every day his memory got worse. The doctor would ask him each day where he lived and Steve gave older and older addresses until he was telling him that he lived in Ruislip, where he had lived decades ago. He took 20 years off his age when he was asked how old he was.

His cognitive functions worsened – he didn't know how to shower himself and couldn't work out what to do with his deodorant, applying it to his hair when handed the bottle. At times, some of his friends were not sure if he recognised them.

November – Treatment

I came in one day and the curtains were drawn around Steve's bed. The Doctor was trying, without success, to rouse him. Later that day the team started him on intravenous steroids even though AE had still not been confirmed. The steroids had an amazing effect, and I am certain that if he hadn't been given them at that point, he could only have been days away from dying. Following the steroids, Steve became more alert, physically stronger and his cognition improved.

He was still confused much of the time and spent hours trying to train the staff and patients around him. Occasionally he thought he was in New Zealand, travelling, and another time he was convinced he was in a restaurant.

He was then given intravenous immunoglobulin (IVIg) for 5 days. His arms were full of bruises and scabs from where he would pull out the cannulas delivering his treatment. The IVIg helped with his confusion but his memory was still impaired.

He could never remember meeting the Doctor, even though he saw him daily. He couldn't retain for more than a few minutes what was wrong with him. He didn't know what he had eaten an hour earlier, ordering coronation chicken sandwiches for almost every meal.

As he showed an improvement in his confusion, the team decided to move him to a neuro rehab centre. He had a second round of IVIg before they transferred him. This helped less, and in fact, he became more confused and sleepier before the transfer.

Christmas 2018 to March 2019 – Rehabilitation and further treatment

Not long after moving to the rehab centre (and two months after his original admission), the confusion resolved. His short-term memory remained an issue and I was advised to buy him a diary so he could write down what he did each day.

Steve was reluctant to engage with the rehab sessions. He was so frustrated by his lack of fitness that it was hard to get him to go walking or running in the park during his physiotherapy sessions. He hated being tested psychologically as he was aware that he was not functioning at his normal level. He was angry that he was not allowed to leave the centre, without a friend or staff member accompanying him.

Gradually Steve's memory improved. The staff were kind and patient. Not being able to remember his passwords, Steve was locked out of all his accounts and devices. The Occupational Therapist took him to the bank and mobile phone shop so that he could start to reclaim his former life.

One thing that wasn't improving was his seizures. They were getting worse and more frequent. He had another EEG which was videoed and reviewed by the team at St George's Hospital in Tooting. It was decided to transfer him to St George's for plasma exchange. He had two rounds taking five days each. He continued to improve – how much of a difference the plasma exchange made at this point I don't know.

Mid-March 2019 - Homecoming

Steve spent five months as a patient in three different hospitals. His treatment will have cost a six-figure sum. The staff in all three hospitals were amazing. In the middle of March, I picked Steve up from St George's to drive him home. It was an emotional moment.

For the first months of his admission, it was doubtful that he would be able to return to living alone. The fact that he was going back home, independently, was incredible and is a testament to both the NHS and to Steve's determination.

In the first few weeks at home, he had occasional outbursts of anger. It took another couple of months for Steve's personality and sense of humour to return.

A year after admission

Steve's seizures are still frequent but much less so than the 10-20 an hour he was having in St George's. He is still on treatment and has just started mild chemotherapy as an outpatient. The hope is that the chemotherapy will dampen down his immune system and the seizures will improve.

Steve finds crowds difficult, he is more impulsive and less inhibited than before, being quite direct with people at times. These were all traits he had before, but they are now more obvious.

Whether this is due to the encephalitis, or a reaction to a life-changing experience, is uncertain. He has returned to work part-time. He has regained his fitness and just over a year after he was admitted he completed the Beachy Head marathon.

His memory of 2018 is virtually wiped (perhaps a blessing for the months of his acute illness) but his short-term memory is back to normal. He can once again correctly guess the time to within 15 minutes.

About Autoimmune Encephalitis

AE is extremely difficult to diagnose as it can masquerade as many different more common conditions. I have worked in health care for over 20 years and I had never heard of AE before Steve's diagnosis. The first antibody-specific AE was only identified in 2005 so research into the disease is in its infancy. The doctor treating your relative or friend may never have seen a case of AE before - they may not have heard about it. Learn as much as you can about AE and its treatment.

The DOLS assessment

And now it feels right for the (DOLS) Deprivation of Liberties Safeguarding assessments to go in – as promised in an earlier chapter of the book. The ensuing pages are taken directly and almost entirely word-for-word, from two actual DOLS assessments undertaken on me whilst I was in the hospital. I have not edited them at all, so forgive the sheer amount of times that Mr Rhodes is repeated. It might be a little annoying but I didn't want to change a thing. I have to say that I rather love the first sentence, "Mr Rhodes started to present with some signs of "not being right". That makes me smile every time!

It is reported around early September 2018 that Mr Rhodes started to present with some subtle signs of something not being right. During this time he visited/spoke with his GP a few times, due to having some nausea and dizziness, and then a minor panic attack, following which the GP commenced Mr Rhodes on Propranolol and Zopiclone. Then a few weeks later Lisa (a friend) took Mr Rhodes to hospital where he spent the night in A&E due to presenting with acute confusion.

Some initial tests were undertaken, and the results were negative. It was thought Mr Rhodes may be experiencing some anxiety-related issues. However, Lisa informed me there had been some suggestion that he would benefit from some further tests, but he felt it was not necessary and he was discharged home.

Back at home, he continued to have episodes of acute confusion where he was not making sense when talking. He was forgetting where he was and had frequent abnormal body movement/twitching. On 16.10.18 Mr Rhodes went to work although he was advised not to, and once there, colleagues alerted Lisa that he was presenting very confused and so it was agreed that they would take him to hospital, where he was then admitted.

On 24.10.2018 The Managing Authority (Royal Surrey County Hospital) submitted a request to the Supervisory Body (Surrey Social Services) to authorise a deprivation of liberty on Mr Rhodes. It noted that he was presenting confusion, bizarre behaviour, possible hyponatremia (low sodium levels), with a history of anxiety and mild depression.

It was also noted that due to his confusion and disorientation, Mr Rhodes was unaware that he was in the hospital and required to stay there for ongoing investigations. It noted concern for his safety as he wanted to leave, and he did not have the mental capacity to make decisions about his care and treatment.

Since the initial DOLS request, there have been ongoing tests and investigations regarding the possible causes of his change in behaviour, personality, and presentation. The hospital is waiting on confirmation that he may have AE. Mr Rhodes is now on a neurology ward and on 1:1 care due to presenting with agitation, and regularly wanting to leave.

Views of the relevant person

Although it is not possible to know his past wishes it is important to note that prior to his admission to the hospital Mr Rhodes was a very fit and healthy man. Lisa informed me that he would visit the GP only if concerned about his health and had recently started to take tablets for anxiety, which were prescribed by the GP.

I met with Mr Rhodes on 12.10.18 on two occasions. Firstly, with Lisa in the morning and then on his own after lunch.

On my arrival to his bed area, he was lying in bed with Lisa sitting next to him. He was dressed in sports attire. I introduced myself to him and explained the purpose of my visit. Throughout the first meeting, he was calm and pleasant, but it was very difficult to follow his train of thought. When I asked him questions about how he was feeling and about being in hospital his replies were not in relation to the question.

Most of the time he spoke quietly, mumbled and I could only elicit a few words. Most of them were in relation to work, such as The Care Act, Social Care Policy, Counselling and Social policy. Lisa explained that he often thinks he is at work, whether training or doing an assessment. Throughout my time with him, he would drop off, sleep, or rest between our discussions and his legs and arms jerked slightly. Involuntary movements.

He also at times appeared to move his arms around as if he was doing something specific. Lisa noted that prior to admission Mr Rhodes had very vivid dreams and one night he did a whole training session. She acknowledged he reaches out a lot and was recently pretending to smoke a cigarette. Lisa also thought that when he is tired, he mumbles more and is harder to follow. She also acknowledged when he is really thinking he can stutter and have spasms, which she thinks are related to the brain.

I also noted that Mr Rhodes had a range of facial expressions and Lisa noted this too and stated that prior to admission he was always quite facially expressive.

There were times when I was sitting with him and Lisa, that he would appear to wake up and open his eyes widely, and would look around the room. I tried to see if he was aware that he was in the hospital, but he couldn't, however, he said that he had been there for three to four weeks, which is correct. I asked him if he could tell me how he was feeling physically but he couldn't.

I asked him how he felt about staying in hospital, and he spoke of two levels of practitioners. I informed him that it was important to try to stop thinking about work and to focus on getting better and he replied, 'How true is that?' Lisa and I spent time talking and every now and then Mr Rhodes would join the discussion but overall it was difficult to elicit his understanding as to why he is in hospital.

When I met with him in the afternoon, he appeared a bit more alert, still confused but I was able to understand him a little more. During this interaction, Mr Rhodes continued to have episodes where he would close his eyes but sometimes it appeared to be more due to thinking than drifting off, or tiredness. When I explained why I was visiting him and what my role was he held onto the word 'freedom' and explained that he liked freedom. On probing further about why he has tried to leave, I again found it hard to follow his train of thought as he mumbled quietly.

I informed him that I understood that he enjoyed sport and that it was important to keep fit, which he seemed to acknowledge. Mr Rhodes appeared reflective and referred to wanting to go in a new direction. We spoke of the importance of having a healthy work/life balance, which he agreed with.

I informed Mr Rhodes that it was important to stay in hospital until the medical team can get him better, and on asking if he would stay, he looked at me and nodded in agreement. I could not be certain that he understood what I was asking him. He then continued back on needing a new direction and referred to a loop.

It seemed to me that he had a loop of thoughts in his head and spoke of care work. As the discussion progressed Mr Rhodes appeared to become a little more anxious and referred to brushing his teeth and needing to sleep. I explained to him that I felt it was in his best interests to stay in hospital and asked him if there was anyone that I could appoint to support him with this and if required challenge this decision in front of a judge. Mr Rhodes did not reply but closed his eyes. I did not feel it was appropriate to ask any further questions.

Views of the others

Lisa Mallett – I consulted with Lisa initially on the phone and she informed me of some of the information already documented in background information. She informed me that since the initial admission, things had moved on and Mr Rhodes was now on the Neuro Ward with no confirmation of diagnosis. However, an MRI came back as abnormal, although there was some sign of improvement on a later one.

Lisa explained that they are treating him with regards to an inflammation on the brain and he had a course of intense steroids intravenously, and was now on oral medication. She informed me that since admission there are signs of improvement in that he is easier to talk to, but he remains confused and his capacity to make decisions remains impaired.

Lisa explained there have been some issues regarding communication between Lisa and Mr Rhodes's work colleagues, regarding confidentiality and information sharing, and that there is a fine line with this due to the nature of his work. However, she also noted his work has been very supportive, and everyone thinks very highly of him and so he has people visiting him regularly.

She spoke of her concerns regarding his financial situation and how best to go about this, as he will have bills that need paying and as he is not in full-time employment he will not have any money going into his account. After some initial thoughts regarding contacting the suppliers, Lisa felt the best course of action would be to speak with the bank, to see if they would agree to an overdraft. In the longer term, we discussed her seeking LPA (Legal Power of Attorney) to deal with immediate issues.

I met with Lisa on the ward on 12.11.18. We spoke about his general fitness and she explained that he is very sporty and does surfing, tennis and running. She also went on to explain as there had been a lot of ill health in his family, with regular trips to the hospital, he was very proud to be fit and healthy and feels that once he becomes aware of what has happened it will affect him in different ways.

Lisa also felt that when Mr Rhodes is more lucid, he appears to have lost time, possibly a few years. We spoke about how important it was to be healthy and she explained that he had visited the GP when he had these episodes of what he thought to be anxiety and although he didn't want to take meds, he did take it with the idea of wanting to get better.

Lisa informed me whilst Steve has been in hospital he has made frequent attempts to leave and will often have his bags packed but having a walk around the ward can assist him, but he will still have his bag with him. Lisa explained it would be good to take him out for some fresh air but presently is concerned about whether there would be difficulty getting him back onto the ward. She also said that on a recent visit she thought about taking him to the coffee shop but after a short walk around the ward, he wanted to go back to bed and was quite tired.

Lisa went on to inform me that overall, he is being treated well on the ward and she felt that certain possible reasons for his ill health were being ruled out. She explained that they had thought epilepsy due to involuntary muscle spasms were now just waiting on the confirmation of AE.

*** Author's Note – The DOLS assessment is not an easy read for me. Not simply because of the sheer amount of times I am referred to as Mr Rhodes (kidding), but also because it is hard to understand or picture who I was back then.*

It scares me some. But more than that it makes me hugely sad. At other times reading it makes me grateful for the rate and amount of recovery that I have made over the last couple of years.

Home is where?

I was discharged home on March 12th, 2019. Lisa came to pick me up and I recall telling her not to rush, that I would likely be sitting on my bed all day whilst the pharmacy prepared my huge battery of drugs. I had indeed seen a couple of other patients sitting there until 9 pm, still waiting. It turned out however that I was all ready to go when she arrived a couple of hours later. Miracles it seems do happen. When you least expect them too.

On walking through the exit doors I started crying (as did Lisa), as it suddenly hit me that I was free now and that I was finally going home after nearly five months in three different hospitals. We stood there clinging to each other for a few minutes, not quite knowing what to say or do, rather like the traumatised survivors of a train wreck, or motorway pile-up.

I came back to an empty house and a depth of loneliness that I had never before previously experienced – at least not to the degree that I do now. I sometimes go to bed exhausted at

8.00 or 9.00 pm only to be pinned, wide awake for hours and hours. And that is not easy to cope with, I can tell you.

It is over a year since the successful diagnosis and partially successful treatment of my AE, and not a week goes by when I don't feel completely lost to some degree or another. I am single and unmarried. I have no children, and no surviving parents or siblings. Without a close network of friends, I fear that in those first few months at home, following my discharge from hospital, I would have drowned in all the worries about my symptoms; which are very clearly exacerbated by stress.

I am still on a phased return to work and every time I have tried to do more than a half-day, three or four times a week, I pay dearly for it with increased symptoms and tiredness. This is finally starting to change now, partially as a result of time and partially due to exercise and listening to my body when it tells me to rest. I have to be honest having absences never gets any easier, and to this day I am pretty much terrified when they are more than just pauses in my speech.

I am always in mind of a line from The Dead Zone, where the lead character tells his father *"when the spells come, it feels like a part of me is dying inside."* To me, at times, that is exactly what the absences feel like. At other times my heart speeds up and my voice is shaky when I speak. Just for a few seconds. I get quite anxious and to this day it's hard not to wonder if one time I am not going to just drop dead.

And yes, I know that might sound a bit absurd or overly melodramatic, but when you are alone with a disease that you cannot make sense of it truly doesn't feel that way. In the early days of my absences I would feel like I was on the edge of some blinding epiphany, or insight into the fabric of the universe, but over time I realise that I was just looking for an explanation or understanding of what is essentially random white noise.

I would have to say that I am a very lucky and very resilient person however, and in the last year or so I have managed to run half of the Pilgrim's Way Marathon, and even completed the whole of the Beachy Head Marathon for the eighth time. I have swum in rivers, and in the sea (in two countries) and I have even returned to surfing (very badly) in France this summer. I am also back playing tennis but dear Lord nowhere near as much as I would like to, or as well as I would like, but beggars can't be choosers I guess.

The downside (and I am not sure that is accurate) is that I cannot tolerate: crowded trains, buses or planes, big groups of people, small talk, a LOT of the music that I used to love, live gigs, and loud or even sudden noises. I truly do not like being put on the spot and even get really anxious if I struggle to pay for something in a shop or restaurant on the odd occasion. You see, I now feel watched and useless. I have to learn that I can take my time and that nobody will judge me as harshly as I will.

I mention all of this not only for sufferers of the disease, but also for friends, loved ones, carers, family, etc. If you live with, or are caring for someone with AE then do check out some websites for an exhaustive list of potential side-effects. You will likely find specific things like: confusion, poor balance, absences, seizures, insomnia, depression, mood-swings, disinhibition, etc. But you might find, depending on the type of AE, things that you would not have expected. Bear in mind that there are many different types, and whilst I have met only a few people over the years, there are loads of unexpected surprises and challenges that I have heard about. Plus, we need to accept that no two people are ever alike, so whilst I may tell you what it has been like for me...that doesn't mean that it will be that way for you.

All I can say is that I only hope that it may help you to cope being as well informed as you possibly can be.

This condition is apparently quite rare for someone of my age, and so little understood that I find little that can comfort or console me when I get dispirited. I have reached out to people on various support websites but have not found many people who have had the LGI1 type of AE. I am hopeful that I will in time. I don't know just how broad the symptoms can run for the myriad types of AE, so can and will, only comment on the type that I have experienced.

I would not hesitate in recommending that you make contact with the Encephalitis Society if you have questions, as they are a great source of information, advice, research, survivor and family or carer/partner stories, etc. And I sure would strongly advocate getting in touch with them on the days when you, or a family member, just feel a need to talk to someone with a level of knowledge, patience or understanding, that will likely reduce you to tears.

Yes...for me almost every single time I call!

I am very fortunate as a single man to have a huge amount of friends and colleagues that think very highly of me. They are constantly reminding me of just how far I have come and how well I am doing, and for that I am so, so grateful. Whilst friends cannot replace real family they are a definite source of strength, support, and comfort to me.

I suppose that it would have been naïve of me not to have expected changes in my personality or emotions, as the brain is so complex that it is staggering. But there are some things that are new or at least markedly different in me now. Here are a few. I cannot tolerate: violence, comedy, joke-telling, some forms of music, TV, newspapers, or small talk. The list (at times) seems endless, dependent on my mood, level of fatigue, or overload.

My take on year one of my recovery process is this: I am far from 'recovered.' And as I write this particular chapter I have just completed treatment number six of my chemotherapy. Yes I know...ordinarily a treatment for cancer.

Finally, if anyone tells you that they find that they are a **lot** more emotional than they ever were before the illness, believe them! Please. I struggled for the best part of the first year at home with my anger alone. It was really fast to surface and melded with a low tolerance for foolishness and small-talk. I got a few comments from friends who were (and still are) concerned about my irritability and low tolerance towards others.

It cannot be easy knowing me, especially since the AE, but many of my friends have stuck with me. But only, in reality, the ones that still give me that little wriggle-room for having been ill. Or just have an unnaturally high tolerance, or level of patience and forgiveness. There are others that have not had those qualities, and they are now in my past. No blame for that. Is just life I guess. Below is an example of my impetuosity and impulsiveness now. Both recognised traits of an AE survivor.

I had asked a couple of female friends to act as witnesses to my will. That meant we all had to sign the final copy with the same pen, in the same room, etc. I had recently broken some bones in my right hand, having hit (punched) the wall after spilling red wine all over a beige carpet in the house that I am currently trying to sell.

The two friends got quite touchy with me as my writing isn't quite as fluid as it was before I broke it, and they were concerned that if the writing was considered to have been fake, that it may invalidate the will. I was equally touchy and went right ahead and signed it; completely ignoring their opinions. At that moment I was furious at being told to wait…for something that has taken months to sort out anyway.

They went home quite clearly annoyed by my behaviour. Get this though…they both made mistakes on the will, which I then had to countersign to ensure the validity of the final document. They blamed me for that!

I woke up yet again at 12:57 am this morning, for what feels like the thousandth time in the last two years, and was once again, unable to get back to sleep. Here are the reasons why I lay there thinking about my overwhelming desire to sign the will in such a stubborn manner and why I now hate hearing 'no,' or 'you cannot have.'

- I am awake at silly times throughout every night of my life
- I have huge gaps in my memories
- I struggle to remember names – of people, places, films
- I have diarrhoea most days from the drugs that I am on
- I have been on drugs for over two years
- I don't like hospitals but have now spent five months in three different ones
- I hate taking drugs
- I have had six Cancer treatments and that is quite scary
- I live alone and have done for 20 years
- I cannot drive for the foreseeable future
- I hate driving anyway but cannot do a big shop, surf, or see friends who live some miles away
- Surreys' transport system is utter shit! Slower than anything imaginable
- I have my good (right) hand in a cast
- I damaged my Achilles over a month ago and cannot run currently

- I have a pinched nerve in my back, resulting in horrible shooting pains when I get up or sit 'badly'
- I had the DOLS that basically took away all of my choices and freedoms
- I had to sit in front of adults whilst being asked to draw simple shapes...and failing at it!
- My writing became the spidery scrawl of a child...and not a smart one!
- That I was accompanied whenever I was allowed out
- That I was asked to prepare basic meals and serve them to prove that I could
- That I stopped reading and listening to music
- That I have to do EVERYTHING for myself.... every single day of my life

So, having lain in bed for a while alternating between crying and feeling angry whilst going through the above list of reasons, I then tried a warm bath, and then sat in front of my laptop until around 3.00 am. I finally got back to sleep. Perversely, as if the above were not enough, I then had the inevitable, almost nightly shit dreams where I felt like an utter bloody outcast as well as a totally awful human being.

I would be foolish – and a very bad liar - if I claimed that I didn't experience some of the above feelings before the disease, but the simple truth is that it has magnified, intensified, and quadrupled them. Therefore my feelings are much, much harder to cope with. Perhaps many survivors of many different types of disease or trauma feel that they are placed on a faster, less even journey through a complex maze of feelings that they are not sure how to navigate their way through as they seek the exit. Who knows?

It is still notable to me that I cry every single day of my life now. And whether that is the result of the condition, or simply my new personality and AE combined I have no way of knowing. Not for sure anyway. Luckily for me crying is something I can accept having undergone a lot of counselling in the past, and having undertaken counselling training too. Without all of that I think I would have rushed straight to the GP asking what the hell is wrong with me. And maybe asked him/her for some serious medications to go with it. Kidding.

Sufferer - I know that I keep saying this, but you will not return to being the exact same person that you used to be. Fact! I have to ask though, is that necessarily a bad thing? We can all stand to improve ourselves and find better ways to be right? Nobody is set in stone or a 'done deal' surely? Life teaches us constantly. When my friends and colleagues say "you are so much more like the old Steve we all know and love," I almost wince and feel like saying, "What a shame."

You see, I would rather like to be different. In fact, truth be told, I would rather like to be happier!

Now I'm here

Monday 24th February 2020

I was recently taken aside whilst hot desking in a local social care team office by the nearest thing that I have to a boss or manager (Lorraine), and asked if we could have supervision. We had fallen out a week or so earlier and my heart sank a bit, as I wondered if there might not be some repercussions to our disagreement. You never know...even as a bank worker.

The disagreement went something like this - she had been having a serious discussion with a member of her staff team and apparently had thought that I was laughing at her. The details as to why are vague, but bear in mind that I am quite informal and had probably said something to her, rather than let her finish her conversation.

Her tone of voice and facial expression was one of hostility, and the more I find out about myself, the more I realise that I cannot be around another person's anger. I had a belly-full of female anger towards me as a kid. It would balance things out a bit if I made the observation that she can appear intolerant of people at times too, but this is not about scoring points. Just evening out the playing field a touch.

At the time I said nothing, choosing instead to move to a hot desk at the other end of the office. After a couple of hours she came over and asked if we could talk about what had happened. I was still struggling with the hurt and anger (fury) towards her. I believe I listened but would not/could not look at her. Apparently, I told her to *"fuck off and leave me alone"*.

Not a moment in my life that I am at all proud of. She was decent enough to say we could talk about it at a later date. The supervision was that later date. By the time it came around (just over a week later) I had recovered my composure and was aware that I had experienced too many rejections from females to be anything but defensive. I do strive to learn from life.

So, I sat down with my boss (and friend) Lorraine B and we spoke with some surprising maturity. I had decided that I cannot continue going down the well-known self-destruct path and that the isolation I feel can only change if I take a whole new set of behaviours and attitudes moving forward. In that supervision I did not feel fear, or anger, or overwhelmed. I felt like a decent human being getting help from someone with nothing but good intentions.

We talked for over an hour and agreed that I would write a short few paragraphs about my illness, the traits that I presented at work, and how my life had changed since the AE. And she promised that this would go out to all staff in the team. I don't know if it was my idea or Lorraine's but it sure had gone through my mind a few times.

It definitely informed the decision I made that I would go ahead and write this book. It also fuelled my desire to seek its publication. It needs to be out there. Even if I am not a famous writer, sports-person, musician, actor/actress...or anything in particular, I have nothing to lose. Then again fame is only really a set of circumstances added to a previously very normal human being.

I wrote the agreed note to Lorraine's staff two days later and the words flowed quite easily out of me. Just four or five paragraphs but meaningful and from the heart. I then sent them to her to approve. She changed one word and asked if I wanted to attach a fundraising page for a run that I am due to do in May 2020, around the Isle of Wight.

I was really impressed and flattered that the boss of a team of people would suggest/allow that. I added the link and submitted my story. I went into work the following day feeling lighter than I had for quite a long while I can tell you. I sat down next to a colleague and she told me that my story was already out there and throughout the day I have had at least 6/8 people quietly approach me and tell me how brave and inspiring it was that I was able to be so open.

I struggle not to cry when people are really kind to me, and that still applies today (in 2022), as I sit in the window of a local cafe, re-writing this for the millionth time - or so it feels. That day however, was one of the likes of which I had not experienced for some years. More than I care to think about, and most certainly more than I can remember if I am truthful with myself. And I don't know if that is because of the AE, or just my low self-esteem.

It didn't matter that day. I felt more 'visible' than I usually do. Or to put it more accurately, I caught a fleeting glimpse of a reflection of someone real, kind, decent, and loved. Oh, and that feels so very, very good to be able to actually write down, re-read and believe.

I now feel that a door has opened. Just a crack mind...but the light that floods through that crack feels warm on my face. I want to fling that heavy, rusted door open as wide as it will go and bathe myself in that light. Writing that I feel an odd mixture of hope and expectation, but also a feeling of fear deep down in my gut. It will take a lot of trust on my part not to keep one hand on the door and stand pretty close to it - just in case.

I pray to whatever God, or being, or belief-system that I have going on inside of me, that I can simply walk through the door and keep on going.

I want to add here, based on an earlier comment - "I struggle not to cry when people are really kind to me" – a little in the way of an explanation. You see, I get almost completely overwhelmed (at times), since being unwell, by the sheer force of my emotional response to kindness, flattery or even help.

Here is an example. Yesterday (25th May 2020) I got my second lot of feedback from a close friend of mine (Clive) who was good enough to read an earlier draft of this book. I sent him it a few weeks back and we spoke on the phone for nearly an hour. He had read the book, and I got really excited as so far I have had only one person come back to me and her comments were similar to Clive's.

She said that it was great when I talk of my experiences of life and that is where the authenticity shines through. However, like Clive, she asked me if I intended for the book to be about AE and surviving it, or whether it was about me. I reiterated to her that in my opinion, there are three key themes.

- My life

- Childhood and ensuing (and ongoing) self-esteem issues
- My battle with a little known, life-threatening illness

For the next forty five minutes or so, I cried repeatedly as the feedback that Clive gave me was staggering. I don't know if it is the heightened emotionality that a person gets off the back of AE, or if it was simply that I am (was) starting to really hear and value the positive comments and praise that people have to say to me.

If it is either of the two...then I am grateful beyond measure. It feels like I am finally breathing fully again. In fact it feels truly amazing. If this is what trusting people can feel like, then bring it on! I want to be a part of the 'world of humans'. Even if I might have to keep that fire exit door propped open.

Just in case.

Lost along the way

I am adding sections to this book a few years after the initial publication as I have previously mentioned, following a recent experience that I had, which I will also go into in more detail a little bit later on. The date at time of writing now is 28.04.22. So, as you can see it is nearly four years since the disease turned up and decided to live with me. I trust that the timeframes do not get too confusing or jumbled for you. I will do my very best to keep on track.

Why would I be adding to or changing something that had been finished and published? It would be a good question if it has gone through your head on browsing the first few pages. The answer is simple, the AE is not done with me yet. Like many diseases that can affect us, it has some lasting effects. These ongoing symptoms have quite a strong impact on me, from day to day. As they will (and do) for many sufferers, so I feel the need to talk about them now, before you get immersed in the past.

None of us can really live in the past though. Can we? And yet the way a person's past looked, or felt, will have created roots to the surface that keep us anchored, to a degree, as to how, and who we are in terms of our behaviour, feelings, patterns, and responses to life. But enough preamble. Let's get on with it.

It's just that I will be making references to 'absences' and memory loss at times throughout the book, and it is important that you understand what I mean. I should refer to the absences as seizures but I don't. They are an aspect of the condition. Essentially, rather than having full-body spasms as some of you will recognise as a symptom of epilepsy, I simply 'go away' for a few seconds. Sometimes a little longer. In that space, I don't really function, and I am at a loss as to how to adequately describe those moments. So if it is okay with you let us leave it at that for now.

In the last year or so, the absences have reignited. Again, I will cover that in more detail later so don't need to give much detail here other than to say they feel stronger, and scarier than they have in the past. A couple of months back, they really took a leap forward and almost every time I had one, there was the most overwhelming feeling (or presentiment) that I was going to actually die. And NO, I am not exaggerating at all!

The feeling of being under mortal threat would rush through my body and this may sound odd but it was always like the threat was coming from the left. Even now, if I have an absence I will look in that direction, though I know full well there is nothing there. For some reason it is virtually impossible not to turn my head to the left. I do not know why.

My sleep patterns, whilst better than they have been for nearly four years, are still disrupted, and I will wake repeatedly throughout the night. Again, this is fairly typical of AE. The dreams are often negative and impossibly dull and 'practical'. Yes...practical, almost as if my subconscious has no interest in fantasy, or whatever dreams are intended to do. My brain simply doles out practical housekeeping tasks, or worries about the price of energy, or a piece of work that I need to do.

Whilst I am on the topic of sleep, I noticed a fair few weeks ago that I was napping again around 3-4pm in the afternoon. I was getting really weary during the afternoon, so I was going to bed and would sleep for anywhere between half an hour to well over an hour. I wasn't overly concerned but was slightly perturbed that it might be depression creeping in. Not something that I suffer from generally, but I am aware that what with all the health worries...it was a pretty reasonable assumption.

So there you have it - three lots of symptoms that could have pointed me to consider that the AE was still not done with me. But I didn't make the connection, which seems really odd looking back now. There were other signs too, but as they are a daily occurrence, like my huge over-emotionality, I kind of ignored those also. The constant tears, anxiety, anger, and other rides on the roller coaster of feelings that I have (almost) come to accept as being potentially a life-long partner. It seems that 'normal life' can get us so distracted that the plotline blurs and we lose our place in the book, or film and wander off into the distance like a character from a war film suffering shell-shock.

I'm relieved that whilst it has taken me a while, wandering out there in no-man's-land lost and alone, whilst shells and artillery were going off all around me that I have found my way back to the trenches, and got myself some hot food and a bath. It would have been easy to have simply given up. Or been blown to smithereens by a landmine. Easy to step on when you can't see them. Easier still if you aren't even looking for them.

I have some scarring in the left side of the hippocampus of my brain from the swelling now. A brief sentence on that from a website I looked at gave this, "*The hippocampus, located in the medial temporal lobe and connected with the amygdala that controls emotional memory recalling and regulation.*" So that may well push me towards being more emotional than before the AE too, but having spoken with a number of other sufferers it seems that it is a hold-over for many of us.

In fact the word 'labile' was used at a conference the other day and I asked what it meant. Is odd that I had not registered the word before, but never mind. I cut and pasted a definition from the Web and have dropped it in here so that you can take a quick look for yourselves.

"When a person is emotionally labile, emotions can be out of proportion to the situation or environment the person is in. For example, a person may cry, even when they are not unhappy – they may cry just in response to strong emotions or feelings, or it may happen "out of the blue" without warning."

And if you are wondering what it is like to have an emotional world that is essentially magnified by about 50%...well, there I am almost at a loss for words. Other than "bloody hard work!" and bloody tiring! Think about it, you spend a lot of your life awake and moving about. Let's say you get up at 7am every day and go to bed about 11pm, then that is 16 hours of activity. Now imagine you had to carry an overloaded full-sized rucksack, rather than a day-sack that whole time...and you are just about in the ball-park. But only just through the turnstiles.

There are other symptoms that I was utterly in the dark about - or had forgotten about - as over time you lose focus on the past (hopefully) and get on with your life in the present. Also, I have no desire to keep researching, and researching a disease that I just want rid of. Perhaps other people do, but I am not made that way. I do not always agree that 'knowledge is power.'

In truth I struggle to even recall the name or details of all of the treatments I underwent. Luckily there are chapters in the book that give detail - not written by me - of each one, the name of it and its intended purpose. So, if you need to know, or if you are wondering if there are steps, tests, indicators, or something that would help you or a loved one, then please do read on! I will say it a fair few times throughout the book - Autoimmune Encephalitis (AE) can be hard to diagnose, but early diagnosis and a timely treatment has much more effective results!

That is a very well known and frequently stated fact.

Okay, so this chapter has given an outline of how it started for me, and in the last few pages I have brought things up to date, to ensure that you get a full understanding of why this book needed to be done in this way. A few close friends have commented that they always felt I should have done this...but what can you do eh? You can (apparently) lead a horse to water, but it turns out that you cannot make it drink.

I wasn't thirsty back then...but I am now!

The second reason that I include some entries from my journal is that it runs out on Sunday 16th September 2018, the year when I got really sick...and 'disappeared' for a while. At that time I had left for a surfing, sea and sand holiday in France with my friend Lisa. There are some entries where I have clearly been suffering from symptoms that would later become AE such as sleeplessness, headaches, nausea, irritability, etc.

Interestingly, someone asked me just last night what I had wanted to be when I was a child. You know...when I grew up. You would think that most people would have an answer to such a question. But I didn't. I sat there wondering why nothing came to mind. It troubled me. After a while I even started to feel quite self-conscious and awkward. The way that I feel quite a bit of the time when I am around people. The only thing that came to mind (eventually) was, "loved," or at the very least, "visible."

I cannot get that question completely out of my head. It is still bouncing around in there like a rubber ball in a tiny room, and if you ever get to see an old horror movie called Scanners, then you will know that the very worst case scenario is that it might just make my head explode. Every time it pops into the forefront of my thoughts I end up crying. And it is because the real answer is that it has never seemed to have mattered what, or who I want to be, as nobody cares.

Not really. I have felt invisible for most of my life.

I make music, and very few people listen. I have written six other books and very few people seem to buy or read them. Rather like the autobiography, a handful of friends have purchased and actually read one or two of them. And again, I am grateful for that. I have done many, many things with (and in) my life. Good things too, but when I look around everyone seems to have turned away in disinterest, or they are staring down at their mobile phones.

So, If you are shaking your head and thinking about putting this book back on the shelf, well that's okay. I am truly happy for you. I have already paid my dues to the Darkman - my inner critic - and what could be scarier than him? He isn't bothered in the slightest that I have written six books either. Nothing that I have ever done has impressed him it seems. He only gives me his full attention when I fuck up!

I am grateful however that after 59 years and a fairly serious brain disease, I finally have something that I've never had before, Faith. Not in a God or religion necessarily, but in myself. I no longer feel quite so invisible. And believe me when I say that it is more precious than diamonds, gold, or millions of pounds in the bank, or offshore investments.

To me at least.

Words have a power of their own. Some of the statements are taken from diaries or journals that I have kept over the years. Other elements of the book are things that other people, friends, and such have told me. They hold a lot of keys to me finding my way back.

Dark Dreams

I am including some dream elements in this book, as I believe that we learn from everything that happens to us. Everything. The below (very recent) dream has certainly helped me understand what I am going through at this time. Staying open and alert to any signposts or mile markers along the way has served me well in the last twenty years of my life. My advice is always to pay attention.

I just woke up – I have had a pretty lousy night's sleep, and certainly not for the first time in the last year and a half of being unwell, I have had dreams of my feeling faulty, broken, an outsider, and an inconvenience for about the billionth time. I was wide awake at 2.00 am and 4.00 am and had an early breakfast in bed to give myself time to reflect.

It struck me that the last dream segment before waking was set in a graphic artist-type studio setting (I used to be a Graphic Designer some years ago now), and it was filled with large, white drawing boards. The kind that you imagine illustrators may use...or at least before computers took over anyway. In the scene a male colleague has a grand mal seizure and falls slowly to the ground, his body twisting and shaking.

I hesitate to go and help for some reason, but finally move towards the desks where staff are still seated. In the dream it is as if they are choosing to ignore the man's plight. I know enough to bark orders that they need to clear the desks and chairs away, to ensure that he is not injured whilst seizing, but I wake before I can do anything else.

Now I am left with the realisation that my anxiety about my own seizures runs very deep, and is troubling me enough to invade my sleep. It struck me that I am the man in the dream. I am terrified of having a full-blown seizure, and how I would/will see that as the final act of indignity and weakness in the progressive loss of control over my body. If it went that way.

I am no longer indestructible it would seem!

Whilst that may sound odd...there has been a part of me that felt, or at least hoped, that I was invincible. Sure, I am the one in the family who has been in therapy for years, but I had escaped being tarred with the physical ill-health that seems to be liberally sprinkled throughout my family line.

On waking, I felt quite emotional and not just a little scared. Nothing I cannot handle though as this has been consuming my life for a fair while now. What is different today though, is that I saw the absences (seizures) as the dark-man if you like. I don't quite know why he is male, but for some reason that feels right.

Now though I am struck that as a young child I was totally terrified of the dark for a good long while. Throughout my whole early childhood years I had nightmares where my bedroom door would be standing open and I would look up to see the outline of a man standing in the doorway. He had no features at all, just a terrible smooth blank white face.

I had that nightmare many hundreds, or even thousands of times as a kid, and my response was pretty much always the same, huge fear coursing through my body, so much so that I could not shout out. I was unable to move or to speak through sheer terror.

Thankfully, I always woke up from those dreams. But they informed my fear of the dark fully and I slept with a nightlight on for years. I don't recall at what age this fear passed on. But it is back now. Not from some childish fear of the dark but more from a terror of what is happening to me physically. Perhaps there is a very obvious connection to the feeling of being powerless. And if I had to theorise as to why, and what it could be showing me, well then it occurs to me to look back at my family.

My brother, my father, my mother, all lacked assertiveness. I hated that trait and still do to this day...but have also got that fear to ask for things inside of me now too. I am hugely grateful now however, that the brain disease (AE) has taken it away – and I no longer tolerate fools gladly! I am assertive as all hell and back now...but quietly hoping to hit the balance point and not get too annoying. I'm not quite there at the time of writing this I will say however. It takes practice.

I have wondered from time to time about the figure in the doorway. Mostly it sits way back in my mind, and maybe months or years go by without my giving him - or it - any real thought. Unfortunately however, he is back and here in my life. And now he has a name - The Darkman. He represents all those childhood fears.

All over again.

A return to 'real' life

Well, we are kind of done with the more medical stages of the book, where I have tried to give a sense of the impact that AE has had on my life. I trust that it has given greater 'flesh' to the bones of the person I was prior to the illness too. There most assuredly will be more challenges ahead, things that I am sure I could never in a million years have considered.

So if we can learn from someone else's experiences, and I do not know that we can - then pay close attention! Many of the things I talk about will affect you – if you are a human. I will talk about how AE has changed or affected me...whichever term fits best. To do that I need to tell you just a little bit more about myself.

Oh, the urge to type "sorry" there was kind of big...briefly!

I have always had a job...well at least as soon as I hit an age where it was legal to have one anyway. If there was one way back in the seventies. I went out and got myself a paper round when I was twelve years old. There were always records and gig tickets to buy, or a girlfriend to take out. I mention this just to evidence that I have a pretty solid work ethic.

It was in fact one of the only things that my father ever praised me for - without my fishing for it too. I know that I have mentioned this already in the book (I think) but my father was most certainly not disposed to any form of unnecessary displays of affection, approval, praise, physical touch. The list could go on. He was from Leeds after all. A true Yorkshireman. But let's not see that as an excuse or get-out eh?

Right before I got ill I was working in a mixture of roles. One of which was as a bank (sessional) trainer within Social Care. Which I really enjoyed. One of the reasons being that I have had years of positive feedback and evaluations, often stating that I make learning fun, interesting, and original. I value such praise highly as we all know that learning can be mind-numbingly dull and painful at the hands of a teacher/trainer who has lost their passion, desire, energy, or creativity.

I am also a bank worker so that I can assist frontline teams with all kinds of things:

- Facilitation of team away days
- Recording of safeguarding
- Some IT courses

- Training of new employees/bank workers

The reason why I am telling you all this (and frankly talking about work is not that interesting to me) is that it turns out that when I contracted AE and was gravely unwell, work was all I talked about. I cannot for the life of me tell you why that is. The mind after all, is way too huge a topic for the likes of me to understand or fully explain. The scientific community, I am pretty sure, would likely agree. Anyway, let's crack on.

I was discharged from the hospital in the middle of March 2019, and I returned to work in May of the same year. Here is the thing, I still have not managed a whole day's work and have been back working for nearly a year - at time of writing! If I get it wrong, and try to work a whole day I pay the price over the next few days, by having increased absences and symptoms.

I still come home some days, and fall onto my bed, or lay on the couch until I can muster the energy to cook or do whatever single people do to get by. Would you believe that having attended an AE conference yesterday (Monday 25th April 2022), I was reminded that fatigue is one of the major symptoms both during and after the disease.

Amazing that I have forgotten so much of what has taken place since Autoimmune Encephalitis turned up out of nowhere and decided to become a lifelong partner.

Oh, I seem to recall that much much earlier in the book I mentioned that I am epileptic now. So, as we speak, I no longer drive a car. Yeah, that sure is an interesting story right there too, as I didn't find out until days before leaving the hospital. It was whilst I was in St. George's Hospital in Tooting that the magic words that I had been craving to hear for so long 'discharge' were finally uttered.

I was due to see my specialist so she could talk me through my daily/weekly medication regime and for us to discuss any further treatments that I might require over the next year or so. As a result of some new-found assertiveness skills that I seem to have 'inherited' either from the disease or maybe just from some deep pool of resources inside of myself, I managed to get her to sit with me for a full twenty minutes.

Believe me when I tell you that was not an inconsiderable feat as a whole 'herd' of specialists had paraded their students past me over the months, like some kind of freak, in a cage. They would deign to spend all of 2-3 (full) minutes on me before inevitably and frustratingly disappearing.

Bear in mind just how busy these folks are and you will see the miracle in those precious twenty minutes that she afforded me and to this very day I appreciate it.

Well, it turns out that one of the drugs I would be taking was for epilepsy. I stopped her dead at that point as not one person - medical or otherwise - had used the word Epileptic. And most certainly not in relation to me. She looked surprised at that and went on to explain that any kind of misfiring of the brain is seen as epilepsy. Go figure! Again...

So whilst I am fairly proud of the fact that I have always worked, and seem to want to continue, the joy of not being able to drive a car has also had a huge effect not only on my working life, ability, etc. but also in many other areas too. Whilst there are some things that I am not allowed to do...there are some other things that I have gained from the AE.

Right now though, I want to come back to, and talk about, the newly found assertiveness that I mentioned above. In truth I am very grateful for the change. Hugely grateful...though certainly cannot claim to have gotten the hang of it - even as I type this. I am afraid that being a little too pushy, or at times outright too bloody honest isn't quite the definition of assertive, but I am new to this...and need lots and lots of practice, before I will get it right. Then again who gets things right all the time? Nobody that I know anyway.

If I am fully up front however, actually asking for what I want and not putting up with other people's shit is really quite liberating. And yes, not just a little too addictive. Not suffering fools gladly is something that truly makes my life easier. The emotional and energetic toll of smiling at, and being nice to every single person, every single day is just too much and I am much, much more comfortable being congruent and honest now.

In the past I would let people get away with murder and bore me close to death. I no longer do! Thank God! The mood-swings, tearfulness, over-sensitivity, and anger however, inform this 'new skill' of mine, and I have had to apologise to people a lot more than I used to.

Oh, believe me when I say that. A lot more. It is no bad thing, saying 'sorry,' as I am most definitely work-in-progress. And you can take that to the bank. Then again, it has occurred to me millions of times over the last few years that this is true of us all.

Surely?

I could not sleep again really early this morning. So rather than toss-and-turn for hours on end, I decided to watch a video on Autoimmune Encephalitis, type LGI1. The research specialist (a professor from Oxford) talked quite a bit about personality changes that AE sufferers usually display. This is the short bullet-pointed list of the three key things that leaped out at me:

- Memory Issues
- Personality changes
- Emotionality (tearfulness)

The ONLY real reason for including this list is because of the phrase that he used at that last bullet point, and I quote verbatim. "Patients often cry at minor stimuli, for example, watching a film." On hearing that last sentence I burst into tears. I am not sure if it was simply from relief, or that I felt in some way 'let off the hook.'

I mention this as it is important to realise that if by some horrible twist of fate, you find yourself experiencing some of the early traits (or symptoms) of AE, or are even being treated for it, then trust me when I say that you aren't losing your mind. Also, your mood-swings may have a seat or trigger in your medication.

Hang in there for as long as you take them...

Oh, and please do not experiment with your prescribed medication timings or doses. Stick to whatever your specialist advises you. Seriously. I have a personal life-long dislike of taking what I perceive to be needless medication, but I have tolerated being told what to do. Almost to the letter. I consider that to be way smarter than taking risks. After all, they took medical training...did you?

To illustrate the amount of ongoing study into the LGI1 type of AE alone, I must just share a statement that the specialist also made in the video, about the use of anti-seizure medications. *"Currently the jury is still out on whether this is surplus to requirements for this condition".*

That sentence I did seize on. Strongly! As I so badly want to get off all of my meds, and my specialist has now agreed for me to do so, as soon as I am weaned off the final dose of steroids.

What I am aiming to do here is write something that will help other people who are struck down with the same, or even a similar disease. If everything that I have gone through - and am still going through, to some degree - helps others, then it might just have been worth it.

I also hope that this book may help friends, family members, and carers, in recognising and understanding that there is a way forward. There has to be a way forward in life I believe, as going backwards is certainly not possible until they successfully invent time-travel. The next statement needs to go on a line all of its own, as it is a highly important one.

'The long-term effects of the disease are reduced significantly from a timely diagnosis.'

Maybe you will shake your head when the next GP scratches his (or her) head and reaches for the prescription pad to address only the individual symptoms that you are presenting with such as: headaches, forgetfulness, disturbed sleep patterns, nausea, odd behaviour, or uncharacteristic anxiety, then please ask them this question - or a variation on it at least.

"Can we consider that this may be a form of Autoimmune Encephalitis?"

Then make sure that you then ask, *"If not...then can we?"* I say this, as unless they do very specific tests, it is very, very easy to overlook.

Never got sick

"I never really got sick as a child. I fractured my hip jumping between two bridges. I had the usual colds and the occasional stomach ache but nothing you could ever call serious".

The above is true. Completely true. But what you have to bear in mind is that not all sickness or illness is visible. There can be life-long pain, discomfiture (or dis-ease) so deep under the skin that it leaves no bruising, no bone breaks, no muscle tears, and no detectable diseased cells. Yet the sickness is there, and causing an agony that lasts and lasts. Potentially for a lifetime.

You could say that it has many faces. It comes (or manifests) in lots of guises. So many in fact that it can take not only your breath away, but also when very strong...your life.

It can turn up dressed as: anxiety, depression, alcoholism, drug dependency, gambling addictions, domestic violence, low self-esteem, sleep disorders, loneliness, suicide, sexual abuse, self-harming, shyness, confusion. The list could go on. And on. And on.

All of the above malaises could be referred to as Mental Health Issues. That would be as good a term as any. A handy 'catch-all', if you like. If we can be happy with that then let's not dwell on names any longer. What we can all agree is that it is often hard to diagnose accurately, and consequently much harder to treat.

And there are likely millions of humans at any given time, in this wide-world who can, or do already suffer from one form or another. In fact, if you think about it surely mental health issues can happen to any one of us? All it needs is the right set of circumstances and Bob's yer uncle. A scary thought eh?

I once (maybe more than once in fact) told my father that whilst I seemed to be the physically healthy member of the family, perhaps I was the one with the mental health issues. I was not suggesting that I was in need of a psychiatric nurse, doctor, or medication, but I was badly 'bent out of shape.'

By that I meant that I found myself unable to hold onto a relationship and didn't really understand why. I did the best job that I could, don't get me wrong, but when love would come along, I would - over time - feel so utterly threatened, defensive and totally uncomfortable in my own skin that I would find the exits and eventually have to run.

I rather think now that it was more that I was the 'keeper of the ghosts' within the family. I was the 'watcher' and the casualty of all the accumulated family sicknesses. I was always the one who would stand at the bedsides of loved ones in hospital, or observe the pain, the anger, the arguments, the closed (or slammed) doors, and the sudden swings or shifts of mood, temper, and temperament within my family setting.

Do you know what I realised after years and years of this? I keep or kept mental notes. I wasn't asked to but it seems that I did. A little dark part of my brain (possibly the Darkman side of things) just pushes its hat way back on its head, licks the pencil tip, and makes reams of detailed notes.

It leaves those notes right up there tacked to the fridge door and I glance at them when I go to get milk, or butter, or cheese slices. Some of the notes fill me with shame when I think of them. If it is possible to feel shame on another person's behalf that is. I will give you an example of one.

My father told me years ago that my mother did not enjoy sex. I personally suspect that she was abused as a child in some way, or enough ways, to result in this fear, phobia...dislike. He recounted to me once how she had such bad eczema on her hands that for quite a long while, early in their marriage, she had to wear white cotton gloves to protect them.

Likely a result of her childhood in my rather humble opinion. Therefore she had a physical manifestation of her deep-seated traumas. We should be able to grasp life, and hold it in our hands, to touch it and savour the feel. But no. Not for my mum. She told me a lot about her family and how she was treated when she was a child, by her own mother. Who, by the way, was a vile, vile human being. Fact!

The upshot of her huge emotional discomfort was that it communicated its way 'out' into the ethers, and with my highly-tuned antennae for emotions, I picked it up as powerfully as any transmitter in the universe possibly could. So, whenever a nude scene, or sex scene, came on the television - as a child, and throughout my teens - the very air in the room seemed to thicken and freeze.

To the point when at times, it was physically hard to breathe. And when (or if) you did manage to breathe out, you could see your breath. Almost as if you had stepped outside into minus zero temperatures. It was virtually impossible to simply stay in the room in fact, as the tension and embarrassment was that strongly and hideously palpable.

One day recently, I went to the fridge to grab a snack and I found one of those 'notes' tacked up on the fridge door. It was written in that sprawling handwriting that the Darkman favours so much. I tore it down, crumpled it up and then burned it at the end of the garden. And not for the first time either.

As a consequence of the above, I have learned to keep the world of intimacy – and no, I don't mean just sexual - safely at arm's length. Touch, flattery, kindness, and just being silent for anything more than a few seconds at a time with another person can result in my wanting to literally crawl out of my own skin.

I believe that memory has an infinite capacity to store information. Whether we want it to or not. And it goes ahead without even asking. Much of that function is healthy, as we are creatures that need to learn and adapt constantly in order to survive and thrive. Maybe a little less so, in these days of mobile phones, cars, and endless safety measures designed to keep us all wrapped up safe and beyond harm.

The truth is the whole planet is pretty much geared that way. You ever wonder how certain plants or trees, or animals seem to be able to produce poisons or induce rashes, or stings, to keep predators at bay? Yet these same flowers, cacti, trees, bushes, thrive and look so deceptively beautiful and are immune to what they themselves produce.

Anyway...I digress. Like many people, I have the ambition to be happier in this life of mine. I would like to feel lighter or more content and comfortable in my own skin too. Yet I seem a long, long way off from realising that ambition, especially after having Autoimmune Encephalitis. I have often wondered how to go about shedding the past, rather like a lizard or a snake sheds their skin.

I have had a lot of therapy and I feel that I have worked hard to rid myself of all the disturbance and turbulence of my past. Yet, I am still troubled by something...and I cannot see its face. Yes, it is the face that I need to see. The face of what, or who, I could not for the life of me say...but it seems to be just that, a face.

I struggle at times - in the past, hugely - not to feel a wave of massive, defensive anger towards others when I feel that my needs may not be met, or that I will be overlooked again. I watch to see if they will (or won't) be and even when I just perceive (and it is very important to hear that word 'perceive') that they won't, I pull the fuck away and quickly. Nowadays - since the AE - I go from calm to anger in the blink of an eye.

Oh, and I need to be very clear on this...I watch every single person around me so closely that it would take your breath away. And I don't miss a single thing. My belief is that I do not deserve (for some reason that I cannot see) to be loved. Or to be a little more lenient - that may be more accurate - it seems that I am not wired to accept, or process love.

I wonder what it is that I am missing. Is it something that everyone (but me) seems to have? Rather like a charging point, or socket...that sits somewhere at the base of the spine. I raise up my shirt and turn every which way, but try as I might I cannot see it in a mirror. It makes no difference how the mirror is positioned, or angled. I simply cannot seem to see it, find it, or feel it.

My single status - I have come to believe - stems from this belief, as I can't risk my sensitivity to others appearing, with someone (anyone) who will lose interest, or who is just humouring me to make themselves feel better, kinder, or more human. My perceptions are so badly skewed in this area and at times, I feel autistic in trying to make sense of my responses to other people. I am deeply aware of this over-sensitivity and work on trying to lessen it, each and every single day of my life.

A friend said to me just last Sunday, that I am always incredibly hard on myself. He was right. I have heard that many times. I have heard that from almost everyone who knows me, in fact. The only change is that I have started to hear it for what it is. I keep coming back to one single sentence and it strikes me as a plausible reason for everything. 'I just don't feel loveable.'

If you have ever seen the film, The Dead Zone, which was based on one of Stephen King's finest books, the below account may resonate with you. Maybe in that cold, slightly alone place deep down inside of you that desperately needs warmth and light. Christopher Walken plays a teacher who is involved in a horrific car crash. He is comatose for five years. On coming round in hospital, he is told that the woman he loved is now married and has moved on with her life. His mother says, *"cast her from your thoughts, John."*

For him it seems like only a single day has passed. He turns away from her, puts his hands over his head and starts to cry. I have wondered, over and over, why that scene resonates so deeply with me. I am starting to suspect that it is because he lost something that he wanted. Love. It wasn't his fault. Just bad luck. He was in the wrong place at the wrong time, and he got bounced into the middle of nowhere for five years. Left out, whilst life simply went on for everyone else.

In that scene where he states, *"when the spells come, it's like a part of me is dying inside"*. I didn't fully know why it felt so powerful to me, but now I do as it is still how I feel when the absences come. I cannot for the life of me trust that one might just kill me. Oh, I am not saying that there is a part of me that is actually dying (I hope) but it is hard to trust that one of them might just stop my heart dead in its tracks. It may seem, or sound, irrational I guess, but tell that to the inside of my head. Tell that to someone who has never really feared death before, but does now. Just that little bit.

And I am not exaggerating in the slightest that only very recently that fear, and feeling that I am going to die has increased. Exponentially!

In an earlier scene in the same film, the character's old flame comes to visit him in hospital. Christopher Walken's character (John Smith) tells her about the book he was reading to his English literature class just before the accident. It was The Legend of Sleepy Hollow. He is explaining how he doesn't want to be in the lime-light or a 'celebrity,' for being the guy who awoke from a five-year coma.

The line he recalls goes like this: *"As he was a bachelor and in nobody's debt, nobody troubled their head over him anymore"*. She asks him, *"Is that what you think?"* He looks at her and says, in that inimitable way that only Christopher Walken can, *"It's what I want. It's what I want"*.

That makes me cry every single time I watch it. How can anyone feel that the world would be better off without them? Yet I have my own version. It is heavily defended by anger, rage, fear, and loneliness. It looks like this: I am terrified that if I get too close to anyone, or if I let my guard down too far, then that person will die. Or leave. Or simply be pretending. And that feels big enough to me to keep humans way the fuck away! Maybe AE was my most successful and powerful rejection of myself.

Sunday 31st May 2020

I have added the date to this entry for a number of reasons.

- So that you know when this was written .
- So that I can tell you that as I sit down to write this, I am as close to panic/fear/meltdown, as I can ever recall being. I don't know why, but I am.
- As I have wanted to avoid doing this at all costs but know that it would 'avail me naught'.

I just re-read that last bullet-point and I can feel that my breathing has changed and my eyes are welling up with tears. My heart physically hurts in my chest. I just need to *'write this out,'* and I need to be as honest and as brave as I possibly can be. As I sit here, I feel that I have no place to hide at all. I have been hiding my whole life, and today I have nowhere to turn but here. I have a mirror placed behind the laptop screen so that I can see my eyes when (or if) I look up.

When I do risk the occasional glance up, all that I see is the haunted eyes of a complete stranger; someone who is afraid and heartbreakingly lost and so, so terribly sad. In those eyes, there is such intense pain, and a lifetime of wanting to be loved and trying so, so hard to feel worthy of that love. This time though, just for who I am. Not what I am.

I never did anything wrong. And whilst that is a fact, I find myself chanting those words over-and-over. First in my head and then out loud. My head is propped in my hands and I look down at all the scars, and the cuts and the bruises that criss-cross my arms, and it intensifies the pity (make that sympathy) that I feel in the depths of my heart. For myself.

I find myself saying the words "*I never did anything wrong. I never did anything wrong. I never did anything wrong,*" and in my eyes, I see the fear of a child who is mortally scared. He is asking me for only one thing. He wants me to reassure him that he is safe and that he is okay. And I am terrified that I cannot. I just don't know if I am 'enough' to be able to look after him. Even though I am (supposedly) an adult now.

Oddly, today I awoke with the premonition that something terrible was going to happen. I just could not shake the feeling, as I went through the day. I had nice things to do with other people, like tennis in the park with an old colleague of mine and a friend coming over to help me fix up a second-hand guitar but I just couldn't shake this awful presentiment of danger.

Underneath it all I was terribly scared. I truly didn't know where to 'put myself.' Luckily, I have learned enough now, over the course of this life, to have just enough faith in my instincts to know that sitting here, writing this all down may act as some kind of a cure. Well, kill-or-cure anyways. That is what I did, and it was very, very hard to do.

In the course of writing this book, I have started to catch sight of a new person in the mirror. Just a glimpse. Someone who whilst not perfect, (who is?) is so much more adult, real, and 'in-focus,' than he/I have ever been before, and you know what? I am filled with a new warmth and a burgeoning sense of self-belief. Here is the good news, I feel it in my heart. Right where it should be. In truth...exactly where I left it.

This line occurred to me whilst writing the first draft of this book. And it seems not only relevant, but also very smart, caring and intelligent to believe that it is an utter truism.

"The one person it's good to be wrong about is yourself."

The reason for therapy

It is a Saturday afternoon and I have been out all day with a friend of mine. I am home now and the house is warm and safe, yet I feel nervous. I cannot quite put my finger on why. I so rarely can. In the last couple of months, my anxiety about 'downtime' (being alone at home) has increased quite dramatically. My therapist (CBT) wants me to find ways to challenge these feelings. And I am willing to (and need to) as we both believe that the seizures, and, or absences are very much triggered by my moods, expectations, frustrations, anger, nerves, or fear. Pretty much any uncomfortable feeling essentially.

So here I am, doing nothing except trying to put down on paper (screen) what I am up against. But that is like trying to capture in words a visceral fight to the death, and this fight looks bloody already. The foe - the Darkman, as we know him now is virtually invincible. Also his reach extends way beyond mine. He is so fast that I can barely keep up with him, or out of his way.

He gets almost every single one of his punches in and I am reeling in the wake of each and every blow. My nose feels like it is broken and blood is pooling in my right eye. I strike out blindly but am losing badly. And this battle feels like my life depends on it. If I cannot win, or even throw in the towel, I am likely to simply cease to be. I will try to reach deep down inside of myself and see if I can find the words, or some way at least, to make sense of this...but I am scared. Keep that right in the forefront of your minds as you read this. I am badly scared.

"I have got used to being and fighting alone."

No. The above line is a lie! I have NOT got used to anything! I have never 'got used to being, or fighting alone.' Alone is just a default setting. It is what I am most used to. And it is a place where I am far away from people and cannot be hurt. So how come my heart, my very being, hurts so much? I am very badly frightened. And so fucking scared that I don't know what I want to do, or where I want to be right now. Nowhere feels safe.

I tell myself that if I were in a relationship with someone that I truly loved, and who loved me back, I would feel safer, or at the very least more distracted...busier? Everyone tells me that this is a myth that single people believe. I think they say it to make me feel better but I don't feel better. I feel huge anger (at times) at their shallow words. I feel like screaming that they don't know what loneliness feels like. Not when it bites so fucking hard that it draws blood simply just being still for a few hours at a time.

So, my therapist has challenged me to spend the whole of Sunday alone. Annoyingly - or should that be conveniently? - I have made plans to meet up with friends in the evening, so I won't fully meet the brief, but that is okay I figure. I am sure not going to enforce another night alone, simply to meet the brief given by someone who is trying to help me understand this fear. I will spend the day alone. I will try to sit, as I am doing now with the feelings as they arise in my best Buddhist way. I will watch, as, like bubbles seeking the surface, they delicately race up towards the light. I hope to learn something. Perhaps a new way of being comfortable in my skin, my body.

It is funny that when you re-read something that you have written it sometimes seems so patently absurd. The 'challenge' of spending one whole day alone! I have spent hundreds and hundreds of them and now that we are in "Covid-World" it's not even note-able. She was, I suspect, framing it in a way that as I am recovering from a serious illness I (like many people) have to rebuild my faith in my body. The longer I take in this "recovery" phase the more I realise that they are right. I am alone a lot of the time and that has given me time to obsess about my physicality...something I have never had to do in my life.

I must reiterate a line that I wrote at the beginning of my story. It is a line that is quite a few years old but as fresh and accurate as the day it was born. *"I never really got sick as a child. Sure, I had the odd sniffle, cold, flu, a fractured hip, and the occasional stomach ache but nothing you could ever call serious"*.

It seems that this no longer applies to me and that when I do get ill, I pull out all of the stops and in typical Steve Rhodes fashion have certainly not done anything by halves. Not this time. I wonder about the term 'anything for a quiet-life,' and if I will ever be able to embrace just a little (maybe the tiniest bit) of that fabled place.

Who knows? It might just be the one thing that saves my life!

End of the Darkman?

I am just one year into my actual return home (at time of writing) and I know that I still have a long, long way to go. I've said before (many times) that life's a journey. We've all heard and used that expression I am sure. To exactly where however I would not be able to say. It's not like I have, or ever really had, a destination in mind. Does anyone? But people around me say things like, 'back to your old self,' and 'return to normal.' In truth I am not so sure as to what that looks or feels like either. I'm also not entirely sure that I even want to go back to how things were.

It was touch and go a few times (I am told) with my run-in with AE. From what everyone has told me since I came back, and started to process what had taken place over the five months from late 2018, to early 2019, it was simply too much to get my head around. I am re-writing this in 2022 and that is even farther down the line, and I am still not sure what to make of it. It's not like it is a set of ingredients, and I have been asked to make some kind of soup, or hearty casserole. No, this is a human life...mine. So forgive me if this takes as long as it takes.

I will say this though, that is as close to death, or being completely lost to the world of sanity as I would like to get. For a fair while at least. In truth though I have had a few 'near misses' in my life. I have had some very near-drownings as a surfer, and one swimming off a beach in Goa in India having been caught in a riptide with an ex-girlfriend and that was just yards from the shoreline.

It is ironic isn't it that when 'drowners' wave desperately for help onlookers still on the beach, or up on a cliff will often wave back, shake their heads and wrack their brains as they walk away, trying to work out if they knew the person. Truth! I had it happen to me one stormy day in Woolacombe, down in Devon.

I had paddled out one morning in big, stormy waves and should have not ignored the fact that not one other surfer was out. Within minutes I looked up and realised that I had been swept towards some very large, jagged-looking rocks and getting closer by the second. I sat on my board and looked up at the cliff.

There was a lone woman, walking her dog and I waved crazily at her, desperately praying that I could convey the level of imminent danger that presented me now. The woman, however, peered down at me then walked away. My heart quite naturally, and quite literally sank too. However, she must have decided to call the lifeguard, just to be safe, and he turned up in a van after some time! Jeez, but when someone is potentially drowning, you would sure hope that a boat would be their preferred rescue vehicle. A van!

Luckily for me, I had gotten my head down and paddled fiercely, with all of my remaining strength across the rip. After what seemed an eternity I recall looking up and seeing that I was now parallel to the beach. Dry land had never looked so good I can tell you. Somehow I then managed to make my way safely back to dry (ish) land. There was no style to my surfing at all on those final few waves which seemed to break every which way, but the way I would have liked them to.

Looking back, I was certain that I was 'done for' and I will share this with you. In those split seconds, when I thought that I was going to die, I felt the deepest, most intense, and most immediate and abiding loneliness that I have ever felt. I saw nothing but huge, constant sets of tumbling waves, sharp-looking rocks, and a watery grave looming right in front of me.

There was another time when I was a kid and I fell off a gate and landed directly on my head. I recall the scene quite clearly. My mother was talking to a neighbour and I was entertaining myself, swinging on the top of the garden gate. Apparently, there was so much blood everywhere that my Mum was convinced that I would for sure be dead. All I recall is laying on the couch being tended to and wondering what all the fuss was about.

I still have a lump on my forehead to remind me of the incident and used to worry about losing my hair and the lump becoming visible. I no longer worry about such things though. It provides character in fact. Anyone else wondering if falling off a gate and landing on your head might, in some way at least, have contributed to recent events in some way? Head injury. Brain disease? Who knows?

At the time of typing this sentence, I am coming towards the end of six rounds of chemotherapy treatment with a drug called Cyclophosphamide. If you have some time on your hands and are curious, have a search on the Web and have a read of the huge, long list of side effects. It is typically terrifying. Would you believe one of the possible side effects of the cancer treatment drug is testicular cancer?

Whilst I am never really convinced that we can learn from another person's experiences I do hope that if you know anyone with AE, or similar symptoms, then maybe this book will help you understand a little of what they are going through. Maybe you are even the sufferer. And if you are, all I will say is 'hang in there.' Let people care for you. It is all that they can do for you after all, as they will be feeling helpless too. More importantly, ask people to help you...even when you feel like screaming at them to leave you the hell alone!

Oh, also ask yourself what you can, or will learn from the process too. Don't waste any opportunities for growth in this life. Remember that God/The Universe - call it what you will - has a big old spade that he/she takes to the back of our heads when we get way, way too distracted to worry about our health, or pay close enough attention to the little details of life.

Personally, I still have quite some way to go before I am ready to pump the hand of my disease, and thank it for all the things it has shown me; and for the things that I have had to endure every day over the last few years of my life. But I will. Be very sure of that one thing. I will!

Maybe the disease was the faceless Darkman who stood in my bedroom door all those years ago. Maybe he found a face that fits well enough and has been visiting for a while. But we have spent our time together now, and it's time for him to pack his few meagre belongings away in his faded old grey rucksack and leave me be. I don't know if there will ever come a point when I will stop him in the doorway and offer to shake his hand, but you never know...stranger things have happened.

After that though I would suggest that he let himself out, as my temptation some days when I feel really low is to shoot him in the gut and watch as he bleeds out on the floor. To just stand by and let the life fade out of him might just be the one thing that would give me the very greatest of pleasures.

My life has been, and at times still is, quite a struggle. Especially since the AE. On the days when I am tired or have spent too much time alone, I forget to be grateful and just want silence to return. Don't get me wrong, I am not suggesting that I consider suicide but I am human (unfortunately) and sometimes I forget to care about breathing in and out too.

I 'woke up', or 'came to' - or whatever term fits the scenario - in hospital in late December of 2019, with a life-threatening brain disease. One that I (and many millions of people in the world) had/have never even heard of. Turns out that I had already spent well over two months in a hospital in Guildford. Of which I recall not a second of. Other than watching people carol-singing in a corridor sometime near Christmas. Everything else is in the Dead Zone.

Not wishing to digress too much, but I love the breakdown of that word 'dis-ease.' It sure suggests that when we get way, way too ill-at-ease in our bodies we will get a pretty sound and thorough 'telling off.' Often by the universe taking a baseball bat to the back of your head. Figuratively speaking that is. You may be wondering what I am on about here. So, let me ask you a question. If you had (or have) emotional scars inside of you, or patterns of dysfunction, or trauma that stays unchecked or un-exorcised for many years. How might it start to make its presence known?

It's tried gently tapping you on the shoulder, and clearing its throat for so long now that it finally gives up as it is clearly not working. So, it has to find another way. It looks around and picks up a heavy looking, blunt object and hefts it in its hands. Once satisfied with the weight of it, it takes a single, powerful swing at your damned fool head. If you are not very careful that is.

Annoying, I thought that I was pretty highly attuned to myself, and would have believed that I was aware of the small areas of dysfunction inside me, and even the areas that hide away in the shadows...it seem that I wasn't smart enough and the big guy with the shovel (or baseball bat...you choose), well, he still snuck up on me and knocked me into the middle of nowhere.

It seems really odd, fascinating, or interesting that as I am writing a book where I talk about my brush with death or at the very least, life in an asylum, where they look after people who dwell, 'in the middle of nowhere,' the whole world has suddenly been swept - with scary, almost unprecedented speed - into a pandemic situation with the Covid 19 virus.

Now we pretty much all get it. Life is precious. And we had gotten ourselves good and distracted.

So, now I am not the only person (that is how everyone's life feels at times of 'crisis') on the planet, to be in some form of social isolation due to illness or disability. I have quite a few female friends who live alone, so we discuss what it means to come home to an empty house at the end of every single day of our lives. It is hard at times but now every person, in most countries in the world, is expected to stay at home and look after themselves in a specific way, in relation to an illness that can affect every single one of us.

I am (unfortunately) a bit immune system suppressed what with all the drugs that I have taken and the recent chemo treatments so I am being constantly nagged by anyone who knows me not to go out, go shopping or go to the workplace - to be fair, nobody is going into work - apart from all the amazing people who work in health and social care, and all of the essential service like food delivery drivers, pharmacies, food shops etc.

Interesting isn't it? Just how quickly we have considered what is an essential service? Those fat-cat business types in all the capital cities of the world making billions each year for some faceless finance company or another....we could care less about all that stuff and I for one am so fucking relieved!

I have never cared about big business and I know that I am stating my ignorance here, but I am a simple soul who now has got back into contact with the child, and the teenager I once was, with all his curiosity intact. He (I) has an odd, almost overly-simple but clear view of this planet that we all share, and I rather love and value that.

We got greedy. We lost sight of what is important in this life. Maybe some people even lost sight of land and that is a point where your heart skips a beat and all of a sudden you find that nervousness fluttering away in your stomach that tells you that you are in trouble. You guys had better start paddling. You can never tell when the next storm might just whip its way up and head in your direction.

We allowed ourselves to daydream and got distracted but now many, many single people and families around the world are re-evaluating what is important about this brief life that we have been gifted. It seems that a serious illness or even the threat of serious illness, has made us all take a long, hard look at ourselves, and all of a sudden the world seems to have swum back into view with an intensity of colour, sound, clarity, and smell that has staggered many, many people.

The increased silence, the minimal traffic, the empty city streets, buses, and trains, the purer air has forced us to marvel and look at ourselves, to contemplate what we mean in the grander scheme of things. For some folk it sounds to me at least, it is almost like they are doing so for the very first time in either years...or in some cases, ever! This universe is older and wiser than any human being that I know of and it sure doesn't need us to survive. As far as I am aware we aren't required here and we seem to have lost sight of the gift that we have been given.

Here's my take on it. I imagine that the wrapping paper was the gift and we tore that off in a rush to get to the big present inside the box. Now we find ourselves outside in the rain, at night with a torch, scrabbling about in the waste bins looking for it in a fever of near panic. Really young kids might understand that last statement.

All that the universe (universes?) and the planet we live on (we are sharing it by the way) has ever silently asked of us, is for some respect, love, and care...and we are pretty close to screwing that up big time. We never were in charge. That was just our egos talking and they have fallen suspiciously quiet recently.

Only fools have ever believed that in my opinion - we just got sloppy and forgot what was important, which is each other (and every other species on the planet). I have had my own version of that confusion now...and I get to watch and take part in this.

The timing is not lost on me.

Life goes on

I am still struggling to become that person that I can see the vaguest of outlines in the mist. I struggle in fact mostly every day some weeks when I lose my way; which is easy to do when the mist becomes really thick. Over the last week alone I have crashed and burned in the most hideous of ways. Just when I thought I was getting the hang of this life as a human being and here I am on the ground again. My knees are all scraped, dirty, and bleeding. My hands all chafed and cut from where I tried to break my fall. Fuck..Fuck...Fuck. Not again!

Let me tell you why and how it happened. It went like this - I am two weeks out of my final CBT therapy session and feeling better about myself than I have for as long as I can remember. So, you can read that as for the first time in my whole life...at least consistently anyway. I had spoken with a few female friends who have tried a reputable online dating site. So I figure 'what harm can it do?' Plenty as it turns out!

I was on the site for nearly a full two days before the meltdown came this time. Has to be a record for me!

I answered the twenty five minutes of questions that set this site apart from the 'smash and grab' of so many other sites and available apps. I posted half a dozen pictures of myself - mostly in sports gear or pretty casual as I dislike dressing up immensely, and off I went into the threateningly deep waters of 'on the market' for a partner.

The initial shallow waters quickly dropped away smartly after only a few steps, and my breath was pulled from my body by the sudden, frigid cold of the now dark grey/green water. I start to swim, slowly at first, feeling tentative and not just a little nervous. To make matters worse, there seems to be a pretty good rip-tide and I glance back at the beach which is now terrifyingly over 200 metres away and getting farther away by the second.

I wave in mounting concern and distress towards the beach that now looks so very far away and some stupid soul waves back and walks on, perhaps wondering if they knew me and at what party we had exchanged pleasantries. Just as I mentioned in the last chapter.

So, after only a few minutes of scrolling through pictures of females that I cannot see myself being attracted to, or they to me, fear and irritation settle into my heart. I ignore it and tell myself to approach it with a different attitude this time.

Perhaps if I just stop swimming and tread water I will be fine, and get a second wind..

Yes, I have tried online dating before and it is like being in the sea at night. The only light is what reflects back at you off the freezing black water. Naturally it can sometimes be scary, but on occasions also liberating, exciting and joyful. *"Stick with it Steve,"* I tell myself out loud, and my voice echoes back across the flat, cold, and now impossibly deep waters. All I have to do is keep treading water and keep my head up. Do not panic! That is how people drown after all.

It is late in the evening now, so I message four women in all, then fold down the laptop lid and go to bed. I am awake early. No surprises there. Naturally I check my messages and I have heard back from only one of the four women I messaged. But that is a good start eh? The others are silent and their profile pictures stare up at me, seeming to taunt me as if saying 'really, you honestly thought I could fancy you?'

I contacted the woman and heard back from her fairly quickly, which is good, as when I get long silences, I (like many people) read into it as a sign of indifference. It is one of the reasons that mobile technology has changed how we communicate in good ways...and some not-so-good ways. At some point in the evening, even though we had been quite flirtatious by text, I thought 'fuck it!' Texting takes too long, and so little gets said or done. So I called her. No answer.

When she called me back an hour or so later, I was presented with a person devoid of pleasantness, warmth, or even human decency. She was short, terse (the same thing really but I like the word), at times she was even quite aggressive, defensive, and at one point in the 'conversation' even sexist, in assuming me to be like all men, which is definitely waving a red flag at the Taurean bull in me!

It turned out that she was of Asian background and a police officer, which I was deeply impressed by...initially. However, she came across as quite cynical of human nature (as can I be) hardened maybe by the very nature of her job, and perhaps previous relationships. I did my usual thing of trying to keep things nice. In short, I put up and shut up. I pasted a shit-eating grin way up high on my face, which on hanging up slipped away like a free climber on an ice flow. I fell very long and very hard to my usual and inevitable death.

I found this quote from a piece of writing that I had done over 20 years ago. The horrible irony...or reality maybe, is that it applies as much now as it did back then.

"When the blackness comes, I go into complete withdrawal. I get as far away as possible and nobody can come

with me, and nobody can help me. Then I am alone. And only then does the anger come; the fury at the world and all of the hatred and contempt that I have felt for as long as I can remember".

In the space of an hour or so that night I deleted everything that I had ever posted on Facebook. Every single song, thought, positive message, and even sponsorship pages for charity runs that I had done. Every nice thing that I had said to people, or people had said about me. Then I posted something along the lines of - *"Just when I thought the world of humans was even halfway decent I am proved wrong! Every single one of you is a black-hearted, self-centred piece of shit and not worthy of trust. Right now you can all fuck off out of my life".*

I want to state, really clearly here, that this is something that I would NEVER have done prior to having AE. It is clear now, that I was senselessly lashing out and my proofreading friend Greg challenged me and asked *"why?"* Why lash out at friends? Not simply the person who had caused the hurt in the first place. I guess that I would have to say that I am not entirely sure, but the song will go something like this. I am a piece of fucking shit, and only by pushing everyone away, can I stay safe. It is a simple tune. A simple melody...but I have been playing it my whole life, and know it off by heart.

It would seem that the fruit never falls far from the tree eh? Or to put it more succinctly, the habits of a lifetime are not about to pack up everything and leave in a single day. I felt at that moment that I could trust nobody and never would again. Give or take a few expletives that were about as articulate as I could be when I really set my mind to it. I had some more alcohol and went to bed. I felt no remorse. Maybe that would come the next day.

You know what though? It didn't and it still hasn't.

Instead, the next morning, I was smart enough to sit down and write to a couple of friends in the USA who I have gotten to know through contacting sufferers of AE like myself. They, in my opinion, have been through a level of illness that puts mine in the shade. I told them, in brief, what had happened. I knew they would understand the huge increase in emotionality that AE brings.

Oh...and please, bear in mind that the disease affects many sufferers the same - the responses to certain situations. It is a very well known side effect of a number of the many different types of AE it seems. I do wonder if it is explored enough, and talked about enough however. Hence the reason for writing this book in some large measure.

As I wrote to the guys, I found myself asking them (kind of) why I am still attracting broken, needy, angry, or hyper-sensitive people...when it struck me that is exactly what I am! Going on a dating site is rather like an ex-drinker telling himself that as he has not touched a drop of alcohol for three weeks, he never really had a problem in the first place. And after all, what possible harm can one drink do anyway?

It turns out plenty.

It truly takes a huge effort to change. Huge! And a fair chunk of time too. The truth is though, time is one thing that I have on my hands right now. In spades. For that I am grateful. I am also grateful that my self-hatred (yes, the Darkman) which the night before had turned on me with the viciousness of old, was now standing there staring at one bloody fang, that has fallen out of its mouth and is now sitting harmlessly in the palm of its hand.

It glances up at me nervously, not looking quite as sure of itself as usual, and I can barely suppress a big old grin and a nod, as if to say, *"yeah, that is going to happen a lot more now buddy".* And maybe, as it turns and slouches away with its shoulders hunched in an uncharacteristic posture of defeat, I will shout at its retreating form, *"you are losing those big, wicked old fangs of yours and that grip that you have had around my neck. And from here on in, you had better watch your back!"*

Maybe I will surprise him/it though, and kill it with kindness.

...now that would be something to see.

Inside the Silence

Thursday 21st May

Yesterday I had organised to play tennis with a friend of mine (Adrian) at a local park where they have six free and pretty darned good quality courts. They are miraculously still open, even in these Covid 19 times. Mind you...they are outside, so you would have to figure that the risk of infection is significantly reduced. These are early days in the Covid-world just for your information though Dear Reader. So people aren't totally sure that to be the case. Let's hope.

We met up and the weather was gorgeous. Before we started the game I asked if we could try playing just for fun and not get too serious about winning. The reason being that in the past we have both found ourselves filled with frustration if we don't play well enough, and the self-loathing looks up, grins, and turns the screws tightly, quickly, and painfully.

To help us lubricate the process I said, *"let's both say fun out loud at the end of every game as a reminder to not worry about the scores."* That did not last very long. I can barely recall having played and served so badly in one game. In my whole life. Ever. It was almost as if I had jinxed the game by making my earlier statement, and my earlier request.

I don't recall if either of us actually said, 'fun' out loud once over the next however long we played for. Ade can be hard on himself too, but not quite as verbally or visibly as my good self. I wished at the time that I was more like him, but in truth when anger visits there is little awareness of the outer world, or other people. Just screaming white noise!

The inner critic turned the screws even tighter than normal and my fury erupted towards myself, and the world at large spun back into the usual negative, and well-known clear view. I hated myself with such pure and intense heat that I thought the tarmac on the court would melt.

My mind was filled with the following, overwhelming thoughts, *"how can this still be happening after all of the therapy, the years of self-reflection and self-awareness? And worst of all - WHY ME?"* Eventually, having served into the net, or hitting the return of serve way out the back of the court, I was looking longingly at the fence.

I so badly wanted to hurl my racket at it. Then pick it up and destroy it completely. It wouldn't have been the first time that I had thrown an object at something, or broken it into a million little pieces. Not since the AE anyway. I didn't do that however. Instead, I went silent and sullen. But in the silence I found something - something new. Something that has, over a few years now, become hugely invaluable. When I am quiet, there is a change of energy. It is slow and incredibly hard to achieve, as anger is (or can be) a hot energy that wants to consume everything in its path. So being quiet and cool is almost against the very nature of the emotion.

That is what I believe anyway.

It was like finding a sweet, deep down in an old coat pocket, just at a point when you are cold, hungry and tired; standing on a station platform late at night, and praying for the delayed train to turn up so that you can just get home. You unwrap the delicious morsel, savouring the satisfying crackling sound that the wrapper makes as you do. A small flood of saliva fills your mouth. And then you taste it. It is like nectar! It feels like the best meal that you have ever had. Yet it is only a sweet. A single tiny little sweet.

In the silence that ensued that day, I found that something had changed. Something had appeared. And it was focus! And it felt really good. I seemed to calm down, and the inner critic - the Darkman - started to pull away...looking oddly nervous again. Ten minutes later - having won three games in a row - I looked up and the court gate was standing open. It turned out...that he had left. He must have got pissed off at me for not falling into my usual vat of self-hatred, and rolling around in it until I stank to high heaven, and became utterly repellent. I guess that he might return, and maybe a thousand more times even, but he seems uncomfortable with silence. And kindness.

Finally I have found something he does not like. *'Quitter,'* I shout inwardly. *'You fucking quitter!'* I laughed, shook my head, and then served out the set. We finished early as my good friend Ade hurt his shoulder. I think my silence and very evident rage whilst I was losing, had also made him just a little uncomfortable too, but I was happy to stop. It turns out that he had brought a few cold beers with him and we shared them back in the park, laying on the grass in the warm early evening sun.

We spoke about the inner-critic. I wondered out loud how it had gotten so strong. He listened. As he often does. We spoke about my AE and the months that I had spent in hospital. I asked him what it had been like visiting a friend whose mind had deserted him. He looked a little uncomfortable with the question, but answered it honestly; as only a truly good friend will.

He told me what it had been like for him, and how he coped with me being so far away. He recounted how he would talk about his work, his family, and everyday life. I listened - sitting there in the park - but the person he spoke of I had no real memory of. None at all in fact!

Maybe there is a subtle parallel with the real me, the one who lives and grows inside. Maybe he will live out the rest of his life without the need for the rage, the hurt, and the bile-filled, self-disgust. It sure makes me hungry thinking about becoming that person. As if the change looks and smells like the best meal anyone could imagine. Better even than that single sweet. Taking all that positivity into my body and my soul. Maybe that is where the notion of 'soul-food' comes from.

A changed, more evolved, more content, and happier Steve - now there is a person I would like to give the biggest, warmest and longest hug to. Maybe when I get home I will climb up onto the roof of my garage and sit or lay there as the summer sun sets. I might even stay a while and watch as the first few stars come out in the night sky

That feels and sounds pretty good to me. What do you think?

I need to quote something that a friend said to me just last Sunday. He said that I am always incredibly hard on myself. He was right. I have heard that many, many times. In fact I have heard it from almost every single person who knows me. I am sure many of us have.

And the reason for including that statement here, is not to pad out the book, as it might come up short on word count. No. It is because of something that Ade said to me last night in the park. It needs to go into this book as it struck me as smart, switched-on and impossibly perfect.

"Scary experiences leave little scars in my head and my heart. And the scars are permanent. But unless you look closely, you'll never know they are there."

I think that to be one of the most beautiful, sensitive, and poignant lines that I have ever heard. Now there is a man who understands pain and the power that we can give to others if we do not develop boundaries or mental filters.

Low self-esteem can be the loneliest, most brutal place on earth at times. I will say this though, it is nice (unusual choice of words) to know that I am not completely alone. There must be millions, and millions of people who feel the same. At times. I am not sure I fully understand, or even recognise all of the ways that I am hard on myself. But then I think about last night's game of tennis and how miserable, bitter, hate-filled, and furious I was. I felt like the world's worst excuse for a human being.

　　...and it's only a game!

Greener grass

In the early quarter of this year - around February, maybe March 2020 I think, I dug up the whole lawn at the back of my house, with the notion of reseeding it. And this time doing a really good job. You need to know that I have tried planting a lawn at three (maybe even four) different houses previously, and have failed every single time. I even had a guy lay turf for me at one house some years back.

As I have a lot of time on my hands currently - what with not being able to manage full working days, or weeks - I figured let's give it another go. I can't fail every single time right? It would be nice to say *third time's the charm.* But even for a guy who is truly terrible with numbers that would be inaccurate. And not helpful.

Well, I have used three large boxes of seeds already. And all different types that cover dry soil, shade, and even full sunlight. And still nothing. I could use that saying now though...as I have used three boxes of seed. Surely it applies now? Okay, well take a big breath and say it with me then, *'third time's a charm.'* Fingers crossed. Cannot fail again right?

Wrong! Once again I have failed. I have fucking well failed and it kills me. I feel my anger, contempt, and self-disgust stirring restlessly at the sight of the threadbare excuse for a lawn that sits out back. I hate it! It acts as a constant reminder that I have failed and I don't need reminding of any of my inadequacies. I wanted so badly to see something beautiful and lush, well cared for, and satisfying. But no. I see something that is weak, ugly, useless, and pathetic.

Sound like anyone we know?

Yep. It has occurred to me over and over again, that this lawn - or attempt at one - mirrors the view that I have held of myself for my whole life. I still struggle to like myself when I spend too long alone. It is so damned easy to feel forgotten as the 'earth' of my self-esteem is also dry, pitted with rocks and weeds. And not just a little threadbare too. Also, being single and alone too much hardly helps to make it any easier.

What strikes me over and over, and over again, is that making changes in one's life is very hard. It takes time. It takes patience. It takes love. It takes tolerance of all of the changing moods and 'weather patterns' that nature and life throw at it. And just when you start seeing those little shoots of new growth appear and you get all excited, the frost can turn up out of the blue and strip them away. If it chooses to.

Maybe it seems odd to go drawing comparisons between my inner-world and a lawn, but the parallels are staggering to me. We can find hints, clues, signs, messages, or learning in every single moment and situation in life. If we choose to. In fact I am quoting Dan Millman's - *The Way of the Peaceful Warrior* book again, when I state that *'there are no ordinary moments.'*

I could lie to you all and say that I am comfortable alone. But if you have made it this far in the book you will know that is simply not true. To some degree - the same as most folk - I most certainly am for much of the time. But the Darkman is also there, and as we all know, he isn't always that reasonable.

Sometimes he pretends to be me, and steals my phone and then lashes out at people who I care about, and who care about me. He sits back on my couch and laughs at me when I re-read his texts, or his ranting emails that result in pushing people away. Let me give you an example of the Darkman (inside me), and just how charming he can be.

Over the last three weeks, I have taken a lodger into my house. He is (or was) a friend. His name is Laurent and he is from Holland. He is also an outdoors type and a distance runner, so we get on pretty well. However, in the last few weeks staying with me in my house he has seen my anger three times. Hmm, there is that number again...three. Odd huh?

Each time it got worse. To the point that the third time, when we were out walking back from the shops, he made the mistake of suggesting that perhaps my illness had not been real. The result was that on returning to the house I snapped and told him to get the fuck out. I handed him the rent that he had deposited earlier that day (in cash) and watched as he left. I have not seen him since and I felt nothing at all.

At the time.

That situation made me realise a lot about myself. One thing is that I still wanted everyone to like me and I was still trying way too hard to achieve it. Most people do to some extent I guess, but this book isn't about most people. Laurent and I were not compatible housemates. A fact that I had, in hindsight, realised quite early on, at least deep down where the 'quiet-voice' tells us something is not right.

I did not take into account my being hyper-aware of sounds, situations, and people since the AE, which makes tolerating noise or movement that is out of my control far harder than I had ever realised. Nor did I even have a clue as to the possible effect that my new-found, and newly increased impulsivity would have.

Yes, a well-known side effect of Autoimmune Encephalitis is impulsivity. One of many.

The need for me to have a safe and quiet place that I can retreat to has taken me a long time to understand and fully grasp. Ever since I was a child/teenager, I have watched people (mostly family members) very closely, and always from a safe distance. The need for that also comes from the violence, and discord that I experienced throughout those early stages of my life. Hmm. Now that the word 'violence' is written down in black and white it looks kind of stark, scary, and maybe a little harsh?

But let's call it what it is. Let's be fully frank, open and honest if we are going to do this right. When one person hits another...it doesn't matter what the situation is (apart perhaps for boxing or martial arts), it is tantamount to the same thing. When it happens in the home, it is called domestic violence. Has such a nice ring to it eh? The upshot is that I have kept people at arm's length for a lifetime. It has been, and at times still is, a very lonely existence. Safe...but lonely.

However, since the illness I've learned a BIG lesson. And that is that people are important, kind, loving and valuable.

Now, for the real clincher. Take a big breath and hold it for a few seconds, whilst I state this for the first time in many years. If the above statement is true, and with the scales finally fallen from my eyes, then perhaps, just perhaps, I am just as important, vital, loveable, and unique as everyone else! It is tempting to put that last sentence into the form of a question. "Am I not just as important, vital, loveable, and unique as everyone else?" Not sure why that subtle alteration would make a difference. Maybe because it would 'feel' more comfortable? But surely comfort is not the only worthwhile state there is. No sir!

Thursday 28th April 2022

Yes, the above date is correct. Whilst I have been out of hospital over three and a half years now, it has still not sunk in, with all of the work that I put in to be a better person that the final sentence bears any reality in me - Steve Rhodes. It took attending that one-day Autoimmune Encephalitis conference to slam me back into a reality that I had completely forgotten.

In some ways.

You see, I met and talked to people who made me feel fully visible for the first time in…years…forever. I am not really sure which it is. All I do know for sure is that until Monday, after years of talking therapies, workshops, book reading, self-analysis, soul-searching, discussion and rumination on who I am and what I bring to the world. I was still lost. I prefer the term invisible if I am truthful, as it was a word that got used a lot by sufferers, carers, professionals and the like, at the conference; in one context or another.

The whole time I have been searching for something that it seemed to me that everyone on the planet has...except for me. And it is some kind of socket, or input that sits somewhere at the base of the spine, or to one side of the spine. It is the connector for love. I have been raising my shirt, craning my neck to try to catch a glimpse of where mine is. I have taken photos of my naked back, and even they show nothing. Nothing at all.

I had gotten so close to simply giving up the search that right up until this week I was desperate to believe that something was very badly wrong with me still. Maybe the AE had taken it away. But I knew myself pretty well before that episode even got aired in my life.

On Monday of this week however, all of those millions of jigsaw pieces that I had collected over the years got clipped into the right places. One-by-one. Just by standing in front of (and listening to) people who had experienced something the same as me - a disease that had resulted in them feeling like, and acting like I did.

They had an illness that to all intents and purposes left them looking visibly fine on the outside. On the inside of them however it was a different story, or a different picture altogether. Their worlds had been shattered, and put back together as best as possible. I could see every crack, and every missing piece that they were unable to find, or glue back on. And I could hear everything that they said. Everything. I spent a great deal of the day in tears. Unsurprising at best I would say.

Hmm, I am aware that this chapter started by talking about creating a perfect lawn. Or at least trying to. It is not lost on me that if that lawn has truly taken...I would have no idea, as I sold that house and moved away, just over eleven months ago. It was doing pretty well when I left as I spent hours, every day for about two weeks, down on my hands and knees (during winter) pulling out all of the rotting metal, glass, bits of machinery, rocks and all manner of other stuff that made just about the worst foundation for any kind of living thing to grow in.

The parallels to the foundation of life, childhood, etc was not lost on me. I gave that soil love. It is a simple thing...but something that every living thing on the planet should be entitled to. It is not rocket science. Not even close. And I am proud that I was able to do that. Yes. Me!

I moved away from the house knowing that I had achieved something. Quite what though it seems I must have been very unclear on. The absences increased notably just before I decided to move. It was around the time that I had kicked Laurent out of my house in fact. I had been almost completely absence free for nearly a year up until that point.

I was almost totally convinced that I had, or was going to make a full recovery from AE in fact. Not unheard of for the type that I had. For a while I wondered if the stress of moving was affecting me. I had even contacted my specialist around that time to discuss getting my driving licence back. Then the absences returned...and almost without warning!

I had decided to go running early one Sunday afternoon, not feeling entirely up to it if I was honest, but figured that it would do me good. About three miles in I doubled over and vomited. Or as close to as I am able, as I have never been able to actually bring up vomit. I got as close as I was able and stood there, leaning against a fence post feeling utterly wretched. And not just a little scared.

I went home and over the next day or so put into motion a whole set of physical tests that ran the gamut of looking for any possible sign whatsoever of a relapse. The potential with my form of AE is about 25%. So not great odds but not terrible odds either. Those tests, all in all, took nearly a year to complete. There were dozens, and with referral times, different machines, clinics, hospital settings, waiting times and the like, that was pretty good going. I don't think there is a machine I haven't been through, or an organ that hasn't been scanned, poked or prodded at some time, or by one medical person or another.

The results - utterly clear of all possible traces of infection, on a physical or cellular lever...if there's even a difference. The diagnosis was that other than some scar tissue on the brain, the area that governs emotion. I was clear, but that the absences could be non-functional. Meaning triggered by emotions. I wasn't that surprised but still didn't understand where that left me, or what it had given me.

I moved to Arundel in West Sussex and found a small cottage in a side street that within months I came to hate. But the town itself, and the people there, taught me so much that I barely know where to begin. It was so friendly that you had to say 'good morning,' or 'hello' to at least 75% of the population as you walked through the streets.

The oddest thing was that within weeks of arriving there I found myself saying to anyone who cared to listen that in some ways I had come there to 'grow up.' Now, I have no idea what that means in real terms, but maybe again, that doesn't matter. I met a beautiful woman in my time there, who after flirting with her, and finding loads of ways to get her to go out with me, she finally said yes.

She has shown the kind of patience and tolerance to all of the ways that I respond when I feel rejected, or not liked enough that writing each and every scenario here would boost the book to the size of War and Peace. All I will say is that having met someone who seems to exhibit a patience and tolerance for my roller coaster world, I finally realised that perhaps she liked the real me. The Steve Rhodes that lives beneath all of the myriad defence mechanisms and angry, hurt responses.

I stayed there in Arundel for only ten months, but in that time I caught sight of a very different person. I got the odd glimpse of a person that was likeable...maybe even loveable. But there was always something in the way. It was my emotional world. It seemed huge, and to me it felt like that part of me was so badly visible and faulted that I was still ugly, useless and not worthy of kindness and decency. So odd that at 59 years old I still felt I did as a child.

I did what I always do, and fought against it. I tried hard to pay attention to the patterns, to learn from situations that I found myself in, but day after day seemed to run straight into a wall, in one way or another. It was like I was still trying to plant healthy seeds into earth that was corrupted, or contaminated by something. I just couldn't work out what that something was.

I have moved back to Surrey now. Not even one full month ago, and within that time I steered my way through waters that got scarily rough at times. But to complete that part of my journey here, and commit it to paper, it seems to me that I need a new chapter.

...and maybe one not about lawns.

Close to the edge

As I typed the final words in the last sentence I got another of the many sharp and rather painful leg cramps that I have been getting for the last three or more years. I only mention it as there are so many different side-effects to Autoimmune Encephalitis that I need to make a note of them as I go along.

Naturally many of them diminish through treatment and disappear over time. Thank the lord! After all, who on earth in their right mind would ever consider going into hospital and accepting drugs, operations, medications, therapies, and the like, if they were going to come back out feeling just as sick?

But there are other side effects that you may well be left with for a longer period. Maybe even forever. So it would be helpful if I am honest and upfront about them. The main one that I know I have mentioned a number of times, but in subtly different contexts, is the feeling of being invisible, or some variation of that feeling at least. I have sat and wondered about it, and it is hard to put my finger on quite what it is that I am trying to describe, or understand.

But I believe that it is mostly encapsulated in the increased emotionality, confusion, mood-swings, over sensitivity (and that can be to sounds, smells, and people too), personality changes, etc. And it seems that having met many sufferers face-to-face on that one life-affirming day - they had all been deeply affected - but on the inside. In that one area of humans that is not visible to the naked eye. The 'emotional world.'

How I could have lost sight of that I had no idea. Ironic that I use the term 'lost sight of' too eh? Here I am stating quite clearly that the thing that helps us navigate through life safely, our emotions are easy to forget about, or let slip out of focus. Maybe as we go back to the daily stuff, like work, family, routines and the like we just get distracted by too many other things. But also maybe we hope that some of the side-effects will, over time, just slip away.

I know that they did for me for a good long while and I guess that I got preoccupied by life too. Just like anyone else. I could not see all of the 'adjustments' to who I was that the AE had made. I was standing way too close to the picture and bear in mind that it is one seriously big canvas. So I had been staring at the same spot for way too long. With my nose just about pressed up to the damned thing.

Moving away from Arundel and back to Surrey somehow gave me an almost physical 'push' backwards. I stumbled a bit, but oddly, even though I am using this as a metaphor for things, AE can result in loss of balance, and poor coordination, but when I looked up I was far enough away from the picture that I saw so much more. And seeing that gave me greater context for who I was. No point staying stuck. The only constant in the universe is constant change, after all.

Then, late one evening, before closing my laptop I noticed an email advertising and inviting me to an Autoimmune Encephalitis conference in London. For some reason I decided, 'what the hell. I am going to go along.' Not something I might have thought about doing before. But I was, and still am, looking for new things to try just to get back some of my old enthusiasm for waking up and actually getting out of bed each morning.

Oh, I had clicked on a link to a retreat someplace nice back in the summer, but it had been sold out and I never gave it much more thought in truth. I guess what with all the tests that I had been put through, and was still going through over the last year, I kinda figured that was the way to get the right answers.

But you know what? Paying the almost ridiculously small fee for the talks, interviews and sessions on offer throughout the day was worth every single penny! Every single one.

I turned up an hour early, as always, so had time to kill waiting to even enrol, or check in. I went and got a sandwich and came back to the hotel. I sat in the huge, utterly empty hall that was set aside for the conference and ate. I was nervous. I will admit that, and often when alone for hours on end, can never be sure just which way my confidence will go.

Like many people I am sure, I have good days and bad days, or up days and down days. Call them what you will. So, I was left wondering if I would go into my little shell, and not talk to people as has often been the way in the past. It took a fair while before even a slow (almost tiny) trickle of people turned up and they, rather like me, sat away from others, looking somewhat unsure of themselves.

I made myself go and talk to a female who was sitting at a side table eating her lunch and checking her phone and laptop. It became clear she was a speaker for the day, so I went and introduced myself. It turned out that she had been to my house a few years back to take bloods for some tests they were running in Oxford. She was a research doctor apparently. We spoke for a few minutes and in that time I did recognise her.

I want to state as many of the odd little side-effects in this chapter to illustrate my point about AE. One is that sometimes, I take a good ten or twenty minutes before I recognise people that I have not met often, or recently, or frequently. So, I have the odd situation where people will come up and greet me by name and I will stand there probably (definitely) looking utterly perplexed as to who they are, or how they know me.

It is rather like a really thick mist descends for a while, but as we speak and find out where we met and the like, the mist slowly rises and clears and I can snap my fingers and go, "*oh yeah, now I remember you.*" It doesn't always work that way however, and I rather feel that people simply think that I use the AE as an excuse for just being forgetful. But I am not.

Many of the people that I spoke with on Monday quickly admitted that their internal-world had been changed and that they struggled daily with this new, emotional take on the world. Meeting people who had gone through many similar things to myself was utterly humbling and life-affirming. I spent a lot of the day in tears. I sat through each talk 'leaking' almost constantly in fact.

It has been this way ever since 2019. The feelings are not diminishing, or losing their hold on me. Why should they? That I felt, at least for one day in my life, that I was not sitting alone on the world's biggest roller coaster, and that when I find myself trapped in the front car and unable to get off each and every time the cars pull into the station, I could at least look around and see others also in the same predicament.

And yes, there is a saying *'misery loves company,'* but there has to be some variant on that that pithy little aphorism that suggests that having any kind of company, or understanding, and yes empathy too...diminishes the burden. If there isn't...then there should be.

Maybe I just need to be reassured that I am loved too. Who knows? It sure doesn't sound like a terrible notion to me.

There are other traits that one speaker - who was unable to attend so had made a video instead - mentioned that had such a profound effect on me that I cried the whole way through his twenty minute talk, but I am pretty sure (on re-checking) that I have mentioned them all as I have gone through my own account. I think it was hearing that he also felt lost, invisible and helpless, and has fought virtually the same battle as each and every person in that auditorium that affected me so deeply.

Maybe he spoke more eloquently than some others...but then, when I thought about it later, he was one of the only people who was in fact a sufferer/survivor of the illness. And he had referred to something that many others had only hinted at, but not made a big thing of - the emotional impact.

After his talk, and for the rest of the afternoon, I kept pointing out - every time there was an opportunity - that we needed to keep the word 'emotions' right at the forefront of our discussions and awareness when we talk about Autoimmune Encephalitis. I was (and still am) very adamant about that indeed. So much so that at the end of the day I spoke to everyone and anyone who had influence, or authority and insisted that I be allowed to speak at the next conference which I believe is in October of this year (2022).

I am going to keep my fingers crossed that they will remember my rather passionate request and let me do so, as it is the biggest impact for many AE sufferers in the ongoing side-effects or whatever you want to call it. Fact!! - in my opinion.

Letters from the edge

I am including here - towards the end of the book - some emails that were sent to me some time after my discharge, when I decided to go ahead and write an account of my illness. Having asked a load of my friends what it was like visiting me in the hospital when I was 'lost' for over two months I had a hunch that they would make for interesting reading and to give me some clue as to what took place when I was utterly 'out of it.'

I asked that they be as frank and as blunt as they felt able to in order that I get a sense of who I was. Also to give a fuller picture or story than just my words. I also asked that they share their emotions if they were able, as I need to feel more.

Hmm...now that seems horribly ironic that I would type 'feel more' as the sheer tidal waves that are my day-to-day emotions are virtually insurmountable at times. It seems that this state is very typical of survivors of AE. I realised this fully when I attended the AE conference in London. And then some!

Anyway, I have digressed for a while again. Back to the task in hand which was the letters that are coming up soon. I promise. They contain information, details, and areas of the story that are in my Dead Zone.

I have nothing to go on but what they tell me. Some of their accounts moved me horribly the first time that I read them. And they are still hard for me to read now...even in 2022. Really hard in fact. They are also quite beautiful however. They hit me bang-on, dead-centre in my heart, which feels like it has been closed for so many, many years. It is rather lovely to have that feeling stirring inside of me now. It is 100% a case of 'better late than never.'

And that cannot be a bad thing. As long as I don't end up drowning. And as long as I can get off that infernal roller coaster at some point. It would be nice as I sure could use a snack, and I am desperate to use the toilet too.

Letter 1 – from Rod

Hey Steve,

Well, there's lots I remember about your time in hospital. The shock of finding out from Lisa that you'd been hospitalised. I cried that day. My first time visiting you in Guildford. I eventually found the ward you were in but didn't have to look too far for you, as you were standing in the middle of the ward in your underpants, completely un-bashful, and oblivious to everything. You were covered in bruises on your arm - presumably from all the fits you'd been having.

The conversation that day was odd. You were mumbling under your breath most of the time, so it was difficult to understand. Lisa had warned me that you would fixate on a particular subject. Prior to that, apparently, you would just talk about work. But when I visited, you were fixating on surfing, and asking me all sorts of questions about what surfboard I own, where I go surfing, etc.

Which of course, is quite absurd - can you imagine me on a surfboard?

I felt as if you at least recognised me that day, albeit you didn't refer to me by my name. At one stage, I think I heard you mutter Stuart's name, which gave me a glimmer of hope. You were quite sleepy though and drifted off several times during our conversation. I found the whole experience somewhat unsettling and certainly didn't sleep well that night.

On the second visit to you, you were much improved. You were at least able to remember my name, and we talked about things other than surfing. You were still very sleepy though and mumbling a lot. The ward itself was very depressing. Lots of very old guys in the ward, one of whom had lost control of his bowels and shat the bed. The stench was atrocious.

Also, there was a moment of unintended comedy - when I walked into the ward, there was a radio on, and someone was listening to the Radio 2 evening show. The DJ was playing "68 Guns" by The Alarm, which apart from being a terrible song, its triumphalism seemed massively inappropriate for the circumstances at that time. But that did appeal to my rather twisted sense of humour.

I may have visited you a third time in Guildford, with Stuart - but my memory is hazy.

By the time you'd been moved to the respite place in Woking, your personality had returned significantly. It felt more like the old Steve. But you just seemed bored and depressed. You were allowed out for short walks/runs, but I remember you saying that visitors were trying to interest you in listening to music, and you were very much of the opinion that you hated music at that point. You also said you were really bored of reading books. I could sense your frustration at your continued incarceration.

But the next update was that you'd been sent home from hospital. Fantastic news, although of course, that wasn't the end of the story. There was still a long recovery ahead.

Letter 2 – From Claire White

Dear Steve

It must be very hard not having memories of that time - so here goes - I asked Michael for his input too. To start at the beginning. Do you remember that I was running a workshop in the church hall in Reigate and you attended with many of the Reigate team? During the workshop, you seemed a bit agitated and shouted out once or twice.

Initially, I thought oh that's Steve being cheeky but then I realised that something wasn't right and asked you if you were ok. You decided to leave the workshop and headed back to the town hall. I caught you on your bike heading off to Dorking and suggested that maybe you shouldn't cycle – but you did anyway - you told me you had been feeling odd and were having some tests done.

I rang Lorraine as I was worried about you. I think she took you to the hospital the next day as she too was worried about you. By the way, the Reigate team were all so worried too and many of them asked after you the whole time you were in the hospital.

I visited you with Paula once and with Michael a second time in Royal Surrey. On the first visit, you were lounging on your bed wearing a running top and shorts. You were having many absences – and whilst we seemed familiar to you and you seemed pleased to see us, you didn't use our names at all. You seemed to be in a loop talking non-stop about work – I think you thought you were at work – and you said lots and lots about LAS training!

The second time when I came with Michael you had a bag packed on the end of your bed and were having a good try at 'escape'! You said you were getting the bus home and kept trying to leave – as a result, we walked a few times round the ward corridors with you trying to persuade you to stay – again you seemed to know us but didn't use our names – and you didn't want to talk about things that previously we would have talked to you about – i.e. music, gigs, etc.

You didn't recognise that you were in the hospital. We left the hospital questioning whether you had the mental capacity to fully consent to your care at the hospital (sorry... ever the Social Worker and OT, but we were really worried and confused and trying to make some sense of what was going on) and worried about your memory, as you didn't seem to have any recall about your life, nor how you got there.

The hospital too were concerned because subsequently, you had a one-to-one person sitting at the side of your bed keeping an eye on you. I think I brought you some chocolate and you chomped your way through it.

Many people who visited at this time got the 'work' talk and we all became worried that as work colleagues we were reinforcing it – Lorraine and Lisa wondered if work colleagues should step back for a bit in case this was the case. I didn't see you again in Royal Surrey hospital but was updated by Paula who visited you regularly.

I then came to see you in hospital in Woking and by this time you were getting a bit better. I bumped into you in the corridor whilst you were walking and again you appeared to recognise me and ushered me to your room but didn't use my name, so I wasn't sure. We chatted in your room – I do remember that there was no chair, so we had to loll diagonally across your bed!

If I remember anything else Steve, I will come back to you. I hope this is helpful.

Letter 3 – from Kate

Hey Steve,

I wrote this earlier and just as it entered my head - so please excuse any grammatical errors! I am not sure how much of this I have told you before and there are many friends who visited you more regularly than me - but this is MY experience.

I frantically kept asking Kel and Guy if they'd heard from Lisa. It felt like I asked them this every day. Mostly they were waiting to hear. I can't remember when Kel and Guy first came to see you in hospital, but I knew that I wanted to go with them. Lisa had advised us that you might not be up to it. So as Kel and Guy were the priority. I respected your privacy and didn't go.

They were devastated when they saw you - but that's their story to tell.

After that, I was even more concerned and none of us could believe what this unknown 'thing' had done to you. I had seen you in September and you seemed well - apart from you thought something was slightly amiss with your diet and headaches/vision. We sat next to each other at the Indian, and chatted but not much other than that evening.

I remember, Guy had said you must get it looked into. So, when I finally got to see you, it was December and you were in Guildford hospital. Although Kel and Guy had warned me - nothing could've prepared me for seeing you. You looked blank when we walked in. Sitting on the bed, at least wearing your usual sports gear.

I didn't think you had a clue who we were...but you were very pleased with the nut assortment we brought you (Lisa's recommendation). Not so fussed about a music magazine. We chatted inanely for a while, and you chipped in with the odd comment. Some of which were on cue and hilarious - we knew you were in there. Somewhere.

The menu arrived and you stared at it blankly. The man was waiting for an answer, so I helped you read it. I'm not sure if you were struggling with your sight or choosing. I think you tried to prove to me you could read by reading every word on the page. You weren't that sure what you liked. I felt helpless. You were still able to make some amusing comments.

Suddenly you shot up off the bed and started to act like you were presenting something at work. Telling everyone to quieten down, or something similar. The nurses looked up. It was very odd, and awful to watch as you seemingly had no idea where you were. After a while, you walked back sheepishly.

This happened a few times where you looked up and thought you were working. I was deeply upset by this and just seeing you like that. I was unable to control the tears rolling down my cheeks - Kel realised, and we went downstairs for a bit to let you recompose yourself (and me, myself).

You had quite a few absences while we were there, but Kelly and Guy informed me you were so much better! They thought you were not going to make it when they saw you previously. They hadn't told me that before.

When we came back to the ward you had been with Guy for a while - I'm not sure how much you chatted but you seemed very tired. We did not stay too long after that as I think you had had enough. As we left, we hugged, and you said 'say hello to the big man for me' - this was the first indication that you realised who I was.

Not a sound

The notion of writing a book was suggested by my friend Kelly some years ago. I forget quite how long ago it was now, but that doesn't really make much difference does it? I have wondered many times if it is something I should have considered more seriously, but generally rejected the notion as the inner-voice kicked in and asked, seemingly casually, *"Why on earth would anyone want to read a book about you? Who the fuck do you think you are anyway?"*

If you have read all the way through to this point, then that rather cruel, rude and dismissive inner-voice will make sense. If however, you have read this page as the very first one...then you will be wondering who on earth would speak to me like that. Read on if that is the case...but maybe go back to the beginning.

Initially, I considered writing an autobiography about myself as a runner, but that didn't feel right. Whilst it is an excellent metaphor for life, what with the ups and downs, the highs and lows that we all experience as we cover the miles, I felt that by adding the psychology and that human perspective, that I may bring something of far greater interest to the book.

Here I am, some years later, actually doing it. It isn't quite what I expected, and it took a pretty close brush with the Grim Reaper to get me started. It turns out that he is the one person who has clearly heard of Autoimmune Encephalitis, and seems to find pleasure in handing it out indiscriminately, to truly decent people who have done nothing to deserve it. Every person I met at the AE conference the other day had no logical, or reasonable explanation as to how, or why they got it.

I have to admit that the more I write, the more I love it. I hope that this book gets published, and I hope that maybe you buy a copy or two. AE alone is a good enough reason to have written this. The fact that it has a small, little-known name is scary. It needs to be known. It needs to be hunted down and trapped in a jar, and handed back to the Grim Reaper. Maybe give him a slap around his goddamn ugly head too.

Maybe even pass on the message to anyone that cares to listen, that life isn't over until it is over. And, if you have an inner critic the size of the continent of Africa, or South America - like I do, or did - then maybe sit it down and ask it exactly what it wants. Or maybe just tell it to fuck off out of your life!

Sunday 5th June 2022

One last date to go in the book before I finish up. And the reason for it is that last night, whilst laying on my couch, not really sure what to do with myself, I sent a couple of WhatsApp messages to my girlfriend (Yes, I have one!) and re-reading them a little later on opened yet another door to understanding myself and maybe even some of the reasons for the relapse.

I will type them in, word for word here, so that you can see what you think. If it doesn't sit right then no worries, but the more I think about it, the more it makes total solid good sense.

"I am realising why tennis is becoming so important to me. It is because it includes other people, and also that I don't see myself as useless, shit, or 'in the way' when I am playing any more. It is one time when I feel visible, valuable and not inferior in any way at all. So, so very rare and very precious."

I must state that as mentioned in an earlier chapter, tennis (like everything) has been a torture in the past, as I have never felt good enough at it. For my liking. The later text read like this, and it woke me up with quite a start, that even on waking up physically this morning (Sunday), it was still playing in my mind.

"It's odd...just laying here on my couch and listening to some music. It occurred to me that if you don't believe in yourself, then you won't believe that others do either. The extrapolation of that is that if you don't love yourself then you won't believe that anyone else can, or ever will...or really does. And that feels so accurate and true for me."

That's it. Word for word. I kind of questioned it to test that it held water by asking myself if it applied to elements such as *trust*, as that is something that I also find hard to do. I often say that I hate humans. If that applies to me...then that sure explains why I project it onto others. If I start to trust that I am loveable, and have really good qualities, then when that positive reflection comes back...whilst it may challenge me or make me want to take a step back, then maybe I will catch myself in future. After all, why step away from the good stuff?

Oh, one last thing on that...the word trust seems pleasingly interchangeable with the word 'faith' and boy but that is one word that seems to get used in all kinds of settings. But what sticks in my mind is the memory of reading somewhere that there was a theory that faith could even be our 'sixth sense.'

When we think of the five human senses we think of eyesight, hearing, taste, touch and smell...but science no longer agrees, and as per usual is split on a specific or accurate number; not that we need definitives in everything for crying out loud! But think about it. Without faith in ourselves, then surely we are lost? Potentially?

Let me move towards the finishing pages with what seems to me to be the most perfect elements to take us towards the end of any book that I could possibly imagine. I will leave it to some famous people, and writers, who seem far more adept with language than I could ever hope to be. Though, in my opinion, hope (or maybe that should be *faith*?) can keep you moving forwards. Before we get to that though let me take a line from the film, Four Weddings and a Funeral that always, always makes me cry.

"As for me, you will ask me how I remember him, what I thought of him, and unfortunately there, I fall short of words. Perhaps you will forgive me if I turn from my own feelings to the words of another splendid bugger, W. H. Auden".

Stop all the clocks

Stop all the clocks, cut off the telephone,
Prevent the dog from barking with a juicy bone,
Silence the pianos and with muffled drum
Bring out the coffin, let the mourners come.

Let aeroplanes circle moaning overhead
Scribbling on the sky the message He Is Dead,
Put crepe bows round the white necks of the public doves,
Let the traffic policemen wear black cotton gloves.

He was my North, my South, my East, and West,
My working week and my Sunday rest,
My noon, my midnight, my talk, my song;
I thought that love would last forever: I was wrong.

The stars are not wanted now: put out every one;
Pack up the moon and dismantle the sun;
Pour away the ocean and sweep up the wood;
For nothing now can ever come to any good.

I am staggered every single time I watch that scene. I am in complete awe of the ability that human beings seem to have for love. I am also humbled by music, by writing, and by the most touching lines that we are capable of creating too. I have already stated that I am 'staggered' by love so it seemed only right to have included the referenced work at the end of this book. Auden captured something very special in just a few short lines - Emotions.

And they are the one thing that utterly defines, and sets us apart from all other things on this planet. That is my strongly held belief at least.

The book that you are holding in your hands right now might also make you feel something. God but I hope so! Perhaps you will even learn something. That would be good. It would make writing and editing it repeatedly worthwhile at least. I will say this though, I cannot and will not apologise for your responses to what you read here. Nor can I be held accountable for your feelings..or lack of them. No, that is down to you, and nobody else. Learn from them is all that I ask.

After all, 'what doesn't kill you makes you stronger.' It is a popular saying and it feels very right to be going in here now. To draw this book to a close then. I was leafing through a book of notes that I was keeping whilst writing it and found this line that I had written some while back. It illustrates perfectly the changed world of a person who was highly emotional before a rare brain disease, and who is now impossibly so...but not ungrateful for it.

"I have just read this last line in a Stephen King book, *'the wind blew hard all night.'* It made me cry. Copiously. And it is only 6.57 am in the morning."

And one final thought before I put down the book, close the door and let you all get to bed, is a note that I found scrawled underneath the *Stop all the Clocks* poem. It was this.

"Is this poem here because the person in question, that you are so desperate to love, is in fact you Steve?"

It sure would be an interesting question to ask myself. But I shouldn't waste any time answering it, as after nearly sixty years on the planet it would be a no-brainer to simply laugh out loud and say, *"bloody right it is!"* Most likely however, I would do as I am doing right now, re-reading this before publishing it, I would simply start to cry.

Again......

Credits

'For all that was given to me when I was lost and invisible.'

I need to thank one hell of a lot of people who have proved to be extraordinary in the giving of their time, money, patience, expertise, their friendship, and their incredible enduring love for the person who is typing this. If I am honest, as I have tried to be throughout the writing of this book, that is not an easy sentence for me to write. So, here we go then.

To my family: Alwyne (Dad), Joan (Mum) and Stewart (my big brother)...oh and the best dog in the world - Pip. It would have been lovely if I had even one family member alive whilst I was going through this...but they have to live on in my heart, and in my thoughts.

To my friends: I would fail hopelessly if I tried to list everyone that I am proud to call a friend, so if your name is missing from the list please don't feel too hurt, or too annoyed.

Lisa Mallet (my guardian angel), Ali Loughran (always there), Phil Wheeler (my oldest friend), Brian and Ros Eldridge, Adrian Goddings (who understands me), Clive Henn (love you mate), Jim Poyser (The real Boss), Gregory Shushan (my other brother), Lorraine B, Barrie and Janet (so grateful we are back in contact), Paul and Julia, Ros and Clive Barnes, The Barnes family (senior), June Mallet, Luke Stewart (I forget how close we are) and finally Tim Mitra (my tennis buddy).

That isn't even close to being everyone who came and visited me and supported me and who offered me a level of acceptance and love that I am still working towards (and always will be) giving to myself.

Let us never forget the staff (and there are countless) in the hospitals that we have access to - amazingly, for FREE! - with our amazing NHS system. As for the staff: who kept me alive, sane, and fit a big, big thank you!: There are not many names that I can recall as that is one area that is taking its time to return. It may never return in full, but what a small price to pay really. Thank you to all the nursing and ward staff too. The cleaners, the orderlies, the doctors and consultants at Guildford, Woking, and Tooting Hospitals.

I must not forget as well, all the staff in all the clinics and pharmacies that have cared for me, administered meds and blood tests too countless to recall too. Even the ones who after assessing me said *'you seem like you don't really need our input, Steve.'* I always liked hearing that. Thank you for that too.

To my specialist: Elizabeth Galizia a big, big hug. I came to truly value and trust your kindness, patience, guidance, and thoughtful intelligence. And I still do.

To (Helpdesk) John – you are a star that shines bright sir. Thank you for my continued existence and for letting me cry each-and-every single time we spoke. Not that it is possible to stop me anyway. No advice, no judgments...you just listened, which in my opinion, and experience of life so far is a real talent, and a rare skill that is all too often overlooked.

References

- Richard Bach - Illusions
- Stephen King - The Dead Zone
- Washington Irving – The Legend of Sleepy Hollow
- Dan Millman - The Way of the Peaceful Warrior
- W.H. Auden – Stop all the clocks
- The Police – Message in a Bottle
- Kate Bush – This Woman's Work
- The Encephalitis Society – website:

  comms@encephalitis.info
- Bruce Springsteen – lyric quote from The Ghost of Thom Joad
- Four Weddings and a Funeral - written by Richard Curtis, directed by Mike Newell

Printed in Great Britain
by Amazon

81953105R00102